PEOPLE WITH

DEMENTIA

THE FERRARD APPROACH TO CARE

FAITH GIBSON

FOREWORD BY LADY GILLIAN WAGNER

Faith Gibson OBE, AM., BEd., Dip. Soc. Stud., Dip. Ed. is a Senior Lecturer in social work in the University of Ulster at Coleraine. Her other publications include *Do You Mind the Time? Northern Ireland Recall, Foyle Recall, Using Reminiscence: a Training Pack, Dublin Recall* (with Friends of the Elderly), *Ireland Recall* (with Age and Opportunity), *Rooms of Time* (with Cahal Dallat), and *Pain and Pleasure* (with Sue Towers).

CONTENTS

Foreword   Lady Wagner   5

1 Introduction   7

2 Design   11

3 Staffing   13
  Establishment   13
  Management and deployment   15
  Training and development   18
  Supervision   20
  Social workers and
      psychogeriatricians   20

4 Assessment and admission   23

5 Quality of life indicators   26
  Privacy   26
  Dignity   28
  Independence   32
  Choice   34
    Clothing   36
    Meals   37
    Medical care   39
  Rights   40
  Fulfilment   43
    In-house groupwork   45
    Friendship club   47

6 Day care   48
    Rehabilitation   52

7 Domiciliary outreach service   53
    Twenty four hour help line   56
    Inter-disciplinary relationships   57
    Incontinence laundry service   57

8 Shared or respite care   58
    Lunch club   58
    Carers' support group   60

9 Conclusion   62

  References   66

  Appendices
    i   Assessment schedule and
        care plan   67
    ii Daily living fact sheet   70
    iii Case example of
        continuum care   73
    iv In-house group work
        programme   76
    v   Day care application form   77
    vi Day care programme   78

  Index   79

ACKNOWLEDGEMENTS

I am indebted to a number of people who have contributed to the preparation of this description of the dementia services based on Ferrard House. The Department of Health and Social Services Northern Ireland has funded the publication which was first suggested by Professor Mary Marshall of the Dementia Development Centre at the University of Stirling.

Yvonne Bakewell, Assistant Principal Social Worker, Bannside Unit of Management gave unfailing help at all stages while Ferrard House staff patiently answered my questions and assisted me in every possible way. Relatives and residents gave invaluable information and added to my understanding of the impact of dementia on all concerned. Georgina McNeice and Ann Smyth greatly improved the accuracy of the manuscript and Steven Compton, Stewart Morrison and Paul Martin warmly supported the idea that 'Ferrard should be written up.'

Everyone, professionals and consumers alike who are concerned with the development of dementia services in Northern Ireland is immensely grateful to Lady Gillian Wagner OBE, PhD. for her uncompromising commitment to good practice and her willingness to write the foreword.

Faith Gibson OBE
University of Ulster
Coleraine August 1991

I am delighted to have been asked to write the Foreword to **People with Dementia: the Ferrard Approach to Care** because there are so many aspects of the work which demonstrate clearly that residential care can be a positive experience. What better to start with than that over five years four residents were able to return to their own homes and fourteen others to transfer to and benefit from conventional residential care.

To achieve such results collaborative relationships, differential responsibilities and clear lines of accountability are necessary, not an easy thing to achieve. The plea for more information so that people with dementia and their carers are not left to struggle on unaided when early notification and appropriate help could be offered sooner is well made, and all the more tellingly in view of the success of the Ferrard House approach.

Giving residents privacy, dignity and independence and the maintenance of all entitlements associated with citizenship are all rightly seen as of primary importance. But the effort required to put theory into practice is not minimised and the insidious potential of perpetuating a staff centred rather than resident centred regime is clearly and bravely recognised.

Among the many examples of good practice I note with particular pleasure the role played by residents' relatives in a support group which can approximate to a consumer's view. The fact that television is used sparingly and not as background noise is a symptom of the caring attitude of staff. It takes much more effort to find a story or a poem to read or to organise singing than to press a button.

Staff could not support the residents, including those with exceedingly difficult behaviour, if they themselves were not supported. Staff are trained and given supervision and the close supportive relationship of the psychogeriatrician at Holywell Hospital means the staff can cope even with seriously disruptive behaviour.

A sensitive continence management programme ensures the home is odour free and volunteers make regular commitments thus involving the community, both achievements which take a lot of intensive work.

Domiciliary outreach work has gradually evolved from residential and day care developments, adding a further dimension to the capacity of Ferrard House to sustain people with dementia and their carers.

It is ironic that such is the success of Ferrard House that one of its principal aims, ensuring privacy for the residents, is almost put at risk by the large number of professional visitors and students. They come to see for themselves and learn from the creative and imaginative response to dementia by staff from health and social services working together at Ferrard House.

Gillian Wagner
July 25 1991

1

INTRODUCTION

Ferrard House is a purpose built statutory home for severely mentally infirm people which was opened in 1970 in Antrim town, Northern Ireland. It was established by the then Antrim County Welfare Committee and in the 1973 reorganisation of the health and welfare services it came under the Antrim/Ballymena District of the Northern Health and Social Services Board. Following the most recent reorganisation it is now a part of the newly created Bannside Unit of Management which consists of the two merged districts, Antrim/Ballymena and Magherafelt/Cookstown.

At the time it was established as a specialist residential home it was a pioneer in Northern Ireland and was well ahead of most statutory provision in the rest of the United Kingdom. Up until the early eighties it provided conventional longstay care for 31 severely mentally infirm people who were provided with reasonable physical care in a safe secure environment. Little social stimulation was attempted and there was no day care or outreach work.

With changes in senior staff, significant developments occurred so that by the mid eighties although the client group remained the same, Norman (1987) in her review of 14 specialist units wrote of Ferrard

'. . . its role is a combination of assessment, rehabilitation, and longstay care for 'confused' physically active people whose behaviour is too difficult to be managed elsewhere. It has a sophisticated and carefully structured programme of group therapy, individual support and goal planning combined with a quite exceptional in-service staff training programme, and commitment to family involvement in care.'

This present account seeks to describe the continuing evolution of Ferrard as a residential facility, its associated day and outreach services and the well established multi-disciplinary dementia service of which it is a significant part.

The development of a comprehensive dementia service has not occurred in isolation. It has to be viewed within the context of the many changes facing the health and welfare services in Northern Ireland. These factors include the 20% planned reduction of psychiatric hospital beds by 1992 as outlined in the Regional Strategy (1986); the perverse incentive of using public funds to support people in private residential and nursing home care which has fuelled an unprecedented explosion in the number of private sector beds; the managerial reorganisation of the already integrated health and social services, including the appointment of general managers; and the far reaching implications of changes in government policy as outlined in the White Papers Working for Patients (1989), Caring for People (1989) and People First (1990).

Against this constantly changing background, and almost despite it, social services staff have worked persistently and impressively to achieve close collaborative working relationships with health service staff. In partnership they have worked to improve the quality of life for residents in Ferrard, and also to offer a flexible, imaginative and acceptable service to older people with dementia still living in the community and to their carers.

Ferrard House has become widely known as a centre of good practice and many visitors come to see its work in action. The staff have reacted to this distracting attention from politicians, civil servants, academics, managers and practitioners, not with smug satisfaction but rather as an opportunity for critical self scrutiny, a chance to value past achievements, consolidate good practice and formulate plans for future developments.

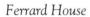
Ferrard House

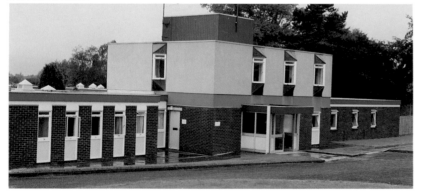

As Norman (1987) wrote '. . . it seems likely that Ferrard will develop into a "resource centre" with a role in improving and sensitising both fieldwork and residential care provision for this client group throughout the authority.' It is this continuing development which is now described. This is not a final statement but a snapshot at a point in time because the achievements are simultaneously consolidated yet dynamic, well established yet ever changing.

The dimensions of residential care identified by the Wagner Committee which were promulgated in *Residential Care A Positive Choice* (1988) and subsequently adopted in the DHSS Social Services Inspectorate's *Homes Are for Living In* (1989) have been used to provide a framework within which the environment, ethos and experience of Ferrard residents are described. The six elusive basic values of privacy, dignity, independence, choice, rights and fulfilment provide the dimensions for ordering the material it was thought important to include. In addition to the in-house description the various extra mural components of the continuum of care based on Ferrard are outlined, because taken altogether they provide a key to a continuing quality of life for people with dementia, and their carers who live in the Antrim and Ballymena area of the Bannside Unit of Management of the Northern Health and Social Services Board.

With the recent fusing of the Magherafelt and Cookstown region with Antrim and Ballymena many of the aspects of the dementia service are now being introduced more widely. Development is continuing apace, the services are not static and although great care has been taken to give an accurate description it needs to be recognised that some aspects may well have changed within a relatively short period of time.

In preparing this account, total freedom was given to visit at any time, to speak to residents, relatives and staff and to observe and report without constraint. Although this account has been checked for accuracy by residential and senior management staff, both the content and views expressed are entirely the responsibility of the author.

The achievements of Ferrard must be viewed within the framework set by the characteristics of the people it serves and its own statement of objectives. Brief identifying details of the 27 people resident in Ferrard on 1 May 1991 are as follows:

- 3 men and 24 women

- average age 80

- age range 66 -93

- average length of residence 2 years 3 months

- range of period of residence 1 month– 6 years

- Number of residents in CAPE categories   Grade C –   1
                                    Grade D –   9
                                    Grade E – 17

- Cape sub scores
  Apathy   D – 7
  Communication difficulties   E – 2
  Social disturbance   D – 4
  Physical dependency   D – 4
  Overall score and rating   E – 20

The Ferrard population is not a static one and residence here does not necessarily mean people stay for life. Excluding short term admissions for assessment or respite, in the five year period April 1986 to March 1991, four residents were able to return to live in their own homes and 14 were able to transfer to conventional residential care. In addition a small number of residents transferred to either a psychogeriatric ward or a continuing care ward in local hospitals.

The objectives set by Ferrard are to:

- individualise all aspects of care

- encourage clients to maintain optimum independence

- maintain familial and community links

- show sensitivity in coping with the dignity of an elderly person

2

DESIGN

Ferrard House at 32 Station Road, Antrim is a single-storey purpose built home, providing accommodation for 31 people in 19 single and 6 double rooms. The front section of the building has a second storey. The home is located within the large Health and Social Services campus based on the Massereene Hospital where a health centre, day centre and adult training centre are also located. Nevertheless Ferrard feels like a self contained unit but it benefits from close proximity to these other services.

It is built on the 'race track' model around a central patio garden. The main corridors equipped with hand rails are of natural brick. Sitting areas, sitting rooms and bedrooms open off the corridors. The lounges and bedrooms have plastered walls painted in pastel matt shades. Plentiful daylight is provided by sky-lights, French windows opening onto the courtyard and large windows in all bedrooms and communal areas.

Floors are covered in vinyl, except lounges which are carpeted. Small light well-furnished lounges are decorated with plants and pictures, many of the local area in earlier days. Furniture is comfortable and functional, looks attractive and corner cupboards and shelves contain ornaments and books.

Bedrooms are furnished with divan beds, combined wardrobes and dressing tables and an easy chair. Duvet covers and matching curtains help to create a bright cheerful atmosphere.

The bathrooms are well equipped. A medic bath and hoist are now little used compared to the popular Parker bath. Some level deck showers are also available.

The dining area is furnished with circular tables which seat a maximum of four people. A wide serving hatch leads to the well planned and equipped kitchen with its adjoining stores and staff dining room.

Staff offices on the front corridor are about to be relocated in the upstairs section of the building. This will free more space which will enable a conservatory to be built out into a corner of the courtyard so providing another informal sitting area as well as opening up the long front corridor.

At the back of the building there is a small two bedroom bungalow which originally provided accommodation for the officer in charge. It has a separate entrance but is linked to the main house by a short covered way and it has direct access to a large garden. This bungalow is now used as a small day centre. The garden has recently been fenced. It has been designed and planted as a reminiscence garden where old time perfumed plants, familiar shrubs, a mill wheel with running water and a turf cart, plough and other farm implements add familiar touches. A half door into the day centre and a small thatched overhanging roof will provide touches reminiscent of Ulster rural life.

Dining room

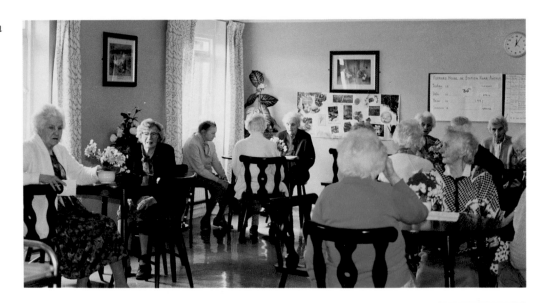

3

STAFFING

Over the years Ferrard has recruited and retained an outstandingly committed and talented group of staff who have been helped to develop practice skills which enable them to work effectively with both individuals and small groups. Staff at all levels are concerned with promoting quality of life as well as quality of care for a client group where traditionally expectations have been extremely limited.

The staffing for the dementia service based at Ferrard consists of:

Assistant Principal social worker for elderly care programme for the new Unit of Management.

Community Manager (Dementia Services)/ Officer in charge, Ferrard

Deputy officer in charge	1	FT
Third in charge	1	FT
Day care worker, senior care assistant (Ferrard)	1	FT

Senior care assistant, team leader	3.67	WTE
• Care assistant	10.92	WTE
Clerical (mornings)	1	PT
Cook	1	FT
Cook assistant	1	PT
Catering assistants	4	PT
Domestic assistant	2	FT
Domestic assistant	1	PT
Laundry assistant/seamstress	1	FT

Gardening is contracted out to a voluntary organisation which functions as a social business and employs disabled and handicapped people.

Maintenance is provided by the works department of the Unit of Management.

The Community Manager (Dementia Services) is also the Officer in Charge at Ferrard. She is increasingly occupied outside Ferrard in helping to extend the service to the recently integrated areas of Magherafelt and Cookstown. Her remit is extensive and includes managing two small day care units, one in Wilson House,

Flower arranging

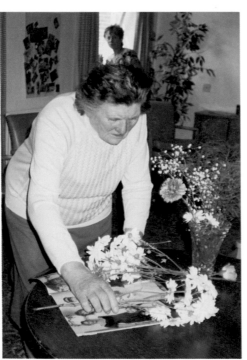

Broughshane and the other in Westlands, Cookstown. She undertakes assessments in the community, at Ferrard supervises the second and third in charge, chairs review panels and copes with the large number of visiting professionals who come to see the Ferrard service in action. The extra mural aspect of the OIC's job is now recognised by attributing 45% of her salary to the community care budget.

In addition to the staff based at Ferrard, the Community Dementia Service also employs day care and domiciliary staff to cover other regions of the Unit of Management. There are two day care assistants working 30 hours a week, one based at Wilson House, and the other at Westlands. A domiciliary worker (senior care assistant), works 35 hours a week in the Magherafelt/Cookstown area.

The Assistant Principal Social Worker who is the Line Manager was an earlier OIC at Ferrard. She now has a broad remit for the management and planning of all social services for the elderly programme of care in the whole Unit of Management so is operationally well placed to ensure that the dementia service is properly integrated with other services and that it is adequately resourced.

A summary of the management roles and tasks shared by the senior staff in Ferrard is given in the following diagram:

THE THREEFOLD TASK FOR SENIOR MANAGEMENT

MANAGEMENT OF STAFF

Setting objectives
Staff supervision
In-service training
Staff selection
Induction of staff
Multi-disciplinary meetings
Team building
Staff meetings
Budget monitoring
Admissions
Domiciliary service
Day care service

MANAGEMENT OF THE PROFESSIONAL TASK

Establishing standards of client care
Monitoring care plans
Evaluating care plans
Monitoring aids
Assessments – individuals
                        – groups
Liaison   – pensions
Relatives support group
Primary worker records
Chiropody

MANAGEMENT OF THE SETTING

Catering & domestic
Maintenance of unit
Furbishing of unit
Ordering & monitoring stores
Health & safety
Budget monitoring
Staff rotas
Entertainment – internal
                       – external

Norman (1987) said 'the staffing at Ferrard House is of exceptional interest for a number of reasons.' These reasons were identified as the OIC and deputy not being involved in routine care-giving because their skills are better used in assessment, staff training, innovation, evaluation and the management of individuals whose difficult behaviour means they require highly skilled personal care. In the years since this pattern has been consolidated further and the responsibility of the OIC broadened to include work outside Ferrard itself.

Senior care staff, one of whom is on duty at all times, are used as leaders of three care teams and they also act up in the absence of senior staff. Several care assistants are capable of acting up as senior care staff. All staff are well placed to secure promotion to other positions and are often successful in doing so. With the exception of one male member of staff, a care assistant, the entire staff is female.

Each senior care assistant heads a team of four care assistants who are known as primary or key workers. The home is divided into three zones, each controlled by a senior care assistant and her team. There is considerable stability in the staff but to provide stimulation, variety and developmental opportunities the membership of the three teams is changed from time to time.

Day staffing, additional to the OIC and Deputy is one senior and two care assistants throughout the day. Usually another care assistant works in the mornings and an overlapping shift is worked from 2.00 to 4.00pm. This overlap period is exceedingly important in maintaining in-house group work and implementing individual programmes of care. There is always at least one member of each care team on day duty in order to provide continuity and the consistent implementation of agreed care plans.

Senior management staff work 9.00am–5.00pm and provide weekend and out of hours cover. Care staff work a 39 hour week on shifts which are either early from 7.50am or late from either 2.08pm or 2.45pm to 10.15pm. Night staff work from 10.00pm to 8.00am. These rotas allow a brief overlap period for the purpose of reporting and handover.

Night staffing consists of one senior care and two care assistants. No staff sleep in.

As can be seen in the table summarizing the staffing establishment, most staff work full-time. This is the outcome of a staff recruitment policy which deliberately conveys the importance of caring for this client group and which seeks by means of active staff training to develop the required knowledge, attitudes and skills.

Senior care staff are responsible for much of the extensive record keeping which is undertaken. Admissions and discharges are recorded, daily reports written, periodic reviews recorded and medical, drug and stock records kept.

Care assistants or primary workers have special responsibility for three or four residents each. Their responsibilities include:

- Care of residents clothing
- purchasing clothing and toilet requisites
- reporting to the senior any changes in physical condition such as changes in appetite, ill-fitting dentures, care of spectacles and hearing aids
- purchasing Christmas presents for the resident and helping the resident celebrate family and other special anniversaries and events

- corresponding with relatives
- keeping wardrobes and drawers tidy
- ensuring an emergency suit case is prepared and available
- escorting residents on outings, shopping trips, social events and church services.

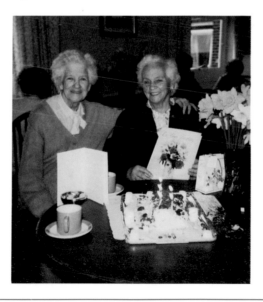

Birthday party

An extensive programme of training for staff at all levels is well established and is used as a means of ensuring that the agreed policy objectives of the dementia service are implemented. It is so central to determining the Ferrard approach to care that it will be described in detail for each group of staff.

MANAGEMENT STAFF

Senior staff are included in general management training within the Unit of Management. A recent series of workshops has included teaching on the management task, models of supervision, the process of staff supervision, leadership and team building, goal setting and individual programme planning. Through such participation the residential staff are closely integrated into the senior management group of the Unit of Management and all aspects of service development including fieldwork, residential, day and domiciliary services benefit as a consequence.

SENIOR CARE INDUCTION

An introduction to:

- staff policies concerned with who's who, duty rotas, leave entitlements and sick leave

- policy and practices to ensure confidentiality

- fire regulations, health and safety at work

- management of medication

- primary worker system, allocation, supervision and management of team

- individual care planning and group work

- administration and record keeping

- safeguarding residents' money and property

- admission, reception and complaints procedures

- appreciation of the day care and domiciliary care services.

CARE STAFF INDUCTION:

This programme is carefully structured to cover who's who, staff policies, the primary care worker system, specific attachments and zoning, confidentiality, channels of communications, fire regulations and emergencies.

The programme combines observation, apprenticeship, set reading, teaching and supervision. It provides a planned induction over four weeks and is subsequently followed up by individual and team supervision.

In the first week a new care assistant shadows an experienced worker and learns about the daily care of residents, the structure to the residents' day and health and safety matters.

The second week stresses observation and reporting skills, and assignment to a primary care team with the assumption of responsibility for three or four residents.

The third week addresses the process of admission and reception, caring for ill residents, teaching, reading and discussion about the care of dying residents.

Week four concentrates on the role of care workers both inside and outside the home including shopping trips, outings, visits to hospitals and clinics, and liaison with other professionals and paraprofessionals.

Periodically a series of in-house topic based workshops are held. Some of the recent topics covered have included age-ing and mental health problems in old people, the impact of admission to residential care, working with aggression, loss, bereavement and death and individual programme planning.

This training programme is modified from year to year according to the defined needs of staff and future topics are likely to include the implications of the community care changes including contracting, coping with acceptable risk and identifying and working with people with dementia who have been sexually abused.

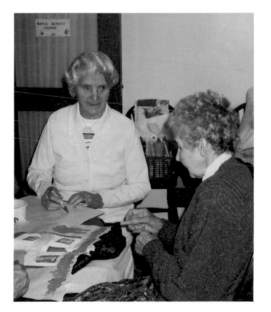

Creative activity

SUPERVISION

All grades of management and care staff receive regular supervision which is managed with formal agenda setting and recording. Senior care staff supervise their own team members and help them to contribute to the formulation and implementation of individual care plans. Care assistants are helped to be sensitive to the needs of residents and relatives and to reflect on the effects the job has on their own well-being and satisfaction.

The senior care staff are supervised monthly either by the OIC or her deputy.

The third in charge meets the senior care staff once a month as a group.

Night staff are supervised by the deputy.

All supervision seeks to combine the three objectives of attending to the implementation of agreed policies, developing and monitoring good practice with people with dementia and their carers and sensitive attention to the impact of the job on the member of staff. Accountability, teaching and instruction, and professional development are all addressed.

SOCIAL WORKERS AND PSYCHO-GERIATRICIANS

One of the significant elements in the Ferrard dementia service is undoubtedly the effectiveness of the multi-disciplinary approach which has gradually evolved. Not everyone concerned is either based in Ferrard or accountable to the same Line Manager. Collaborative relationships, differential responsibilities and clear lines of accountability have evolved over time. All these factors are essential for successful multi-disciplinary work.

The consultant psychogeriatrician with a special attachment to Ferrard plays a central role in the whole service. He is based in Holywell Psychiatric Hospital. Social work for his in-patients is undertaken by hospital based social workers.

The community care teams in Antrim and Ballymena fieldwork offices each has a social worker who is responsible for the social work service for people living in the community who are in contact with the psychogeriatrician and Ferrard staff. They are not working exclusively with people with dementia but have other duties concerned with older people and their families.

Together with other members of the multi-disciplinary team they are involved in assessment, monitoring, reviewing and counselling. Early notification and identification of people with dementia is considered crucial but is exceedingly difficult to achieve. All too often referrals from general practitioners come only at a point of crisis when an immediate and extreme response is required in order to avert a person becoming a risk to themselves or to others.

It is recognised that improved public information and more effective professional education about the nature of dementia are required if early referrals are to be achieved and crisis work reduced. Too many people with dementia and their carers are left to struggle on unaided when early notification would mean that appropriate help could be offered sooner. Miller (1991) raised this crucial issue in saying:

> 'What is important is how do you actually make amenities available to people when they don't know about it . . . They are hard to find out about, information is not readily available. The GP sometimes knows but often doesn't. So you need to have something which is like an information bureau in a railway station.'

The whole multi-disciplinary team continues to address this problem of poor take up of information and late referral. In order to combat these obstacles which are a serious problem even in a relatively small circumscribed catchment area, the psychogeriatrician has introduced an open referral system but he has serious reservations about how effective it is in securing early referrals.

Field social workers are closely involved with the domiciliary care worker and their close collaborative complementary relationships have already been described. In some cases their roles may overlap but on any particular case, separate respective responsibilities are very clearly defined. Mutual respect and parity of esteem for each one's own particular expertise together with a climate of open communication has made good working relationships possible.

Many people with dementia who are being supported in the community have a home help who will be managed, not by the social worker but by a social work assistant. Home helps are used flexibly and imaginatively although their availability is somewhat limited in terms of the hours worked.

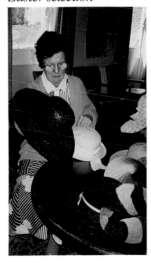

Easter selection

The array of different people involved in any one package of care could become in itself a source of confusion for recipients. Close co-ordination is required. This is only achieved by constant attention to detailed planning, co-operative implementation of care plans and conscientious use of clear lines of communication. The professional carers share common objectives and commitments and the management structures support the implementation of these agreed objectives.

Because all social services for older people, including people with dementia are managed at unit level by one person, an Assistant Principal social worker who was previously the Ferrard OIC, it is possible to have clear accountability across field, domiciliary, residential and day care services. Competing professional interests and disparate loyalties are thereby reduced and a single minded commitment to acquiring and dispersing resources has been established.

Peat loading

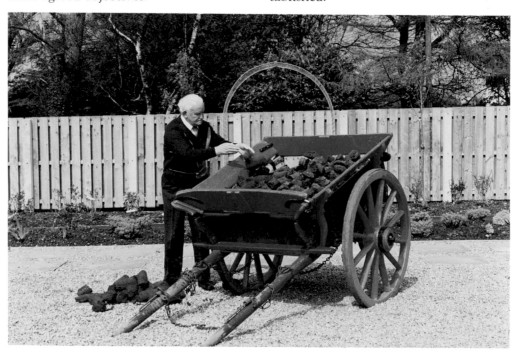

4

ASSESSMENT AND ADMISSION

The policy statement on admission to Ferrard formally sets out the minimum criteria as follows:

1 The client has no (other) friends or relatives who would be prepared to care for the elderly person in their own home.

2 Any community services which might reduce the client's need for residential care should have been considered for him/her.

3 Client is not bedfast or doubly incontinent.

4 Client must be highly mobile without the use of aids.

5 Client is unsuitable for sheltered accommodation, (if available) usually for one or more of the following reasons:–

    (a) cannot get up or wash himself/herself without assistance

    (b) cannot make himself/herself a hot drink without assistance

    (c) and is subject to mental confusion resulting in dangerous occurrences.

6 Ferrard being a 31 bedded unit for the elderly confused it must be highlighted that 'confusion' in itself is not a reason for automatic consideration for Ferrard. Clients being considered for admission will normally be in an agitated state and/or exhibiting abhorrent social behaviour which could not be managed in a conventional unit.

7 It should also be pointed out that where as part of the assessment the social worker deems the client to be incapable of making an informed decision regarding application for Ferrard admission then this must be certified by the client's G.P. prior to the next-of-kin's permission being sought.

A very comprehensive assessment is undertaken of people being considered for admission to Ferrard. A multi-disciplinary team performs the assessment function and a review group meeting every four to six weeks considers the various reports submitted, makes decisions and formulates care plans. (See Appendix 1).

Assessment may be undertaken on either a residential or day care basis. As well as general practitioner, psychogeriatrician, OIC, social worker and domiciliary care worker reports, a battery of assessment instruments is used. Some are well known widely used instruments and others have been constructed by Ferrard for its own use. Careful observation and detailed communication with all concerned are the characteristics of the comprehensive assessment.

Sharing

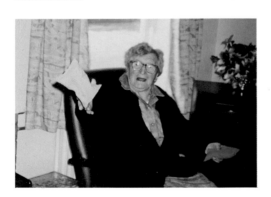

The battery consists of the following:

- CAPE
- Holden's communication scale
- Holden's verbal orientation, personal & current information
- Behaviour rating scale
- Wood's concentration test
- Daily living fact sheet (See Appendix 2).
- Ferrard assessment scale (Administered at beginning and end of the assessment period. See Appendix 3).

The Fact Sheet of Daily Living summarises past habits, interests, activities, preferences and capabilities. It is especially helpful in planning a very finely tuned individualised programme of care.

The Ferrard Assessment Schedule is a comprehensive summary of the present functional capacity of the person and includes descriptive statements covering: mobility: bathing and dressing; use of toilet; continence pattern; spatial orientation, sleeping patterns; communication; social relations; concentration; and memory. The primary care team or the day care worker are responsible for completing this form.

All this information is considered by the review group. Admission decisions are taken and other business transacted. The meeting is chaired by the Ferrard OIC and minutes are kept. In addition to decisions concerning assessment and admission matters, five residents are reviewed at each meeting on the basis of previously circulated written reports prepared by the senior care team leaders. The information reported summarizes the observations and recommendations accumulated by the care team and the day care worker through their contact with the resident. This procedure ensures that all residents, not just problematic ones are regularly reviewed. It guarantees that care plans are kept up to date, relevant and responsive to changing need.

The psychogeriatrician who is a valued member of this group will review medication, advise on behavioral problems and raise other matters for consideration. For example it is this group which considers the possibility of transferring people presently in Holywell to Ferrard or vice versa. The review panel is an effective device for endeavouring to make the best possible use of all the relevant Health and Social Services resources available. By means of careful assessment and disciplined decision making the dementia service is able to provide a continuum of care to meet the changing needs of people with dementia.

A case example illustrating this continuum is given in Appendix 3

Washing up

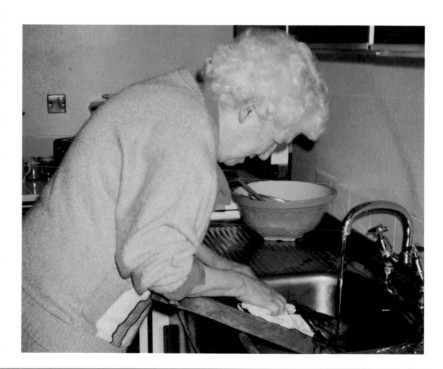

5

QUALITY OF LIFE INDICATORS

The right of individuals to be left alone or undisturbed and free from intrusion or public attention into their affairs.

Over the past eight to ten years, the staff in Ferrard have refused to accept that elderly mentally infirm people deserve any less attention to their basic human needs, rights and dignity than any other person living in residential accommodation. The residents are regarded first as people and only then as people with dementia who may need some additional protection, care and attention.

The design of the building with a majority of single rooms lends itself at least to a substantial extent to balancing the need for privacy and the need for protection. Bedrooms and their furniture are not lockable but every effort is made to respect privacy. Individuals are free to remain alone, or to opt out of group activities if they express such a preference although it is recognised that a great deal of staff effort is devoted to trying to involve residents in sociable activities of various kinds.

The Home with its interior courtyard and recently fenced and landscaped garden affords considerable privacy. At present the garden is overlooked by the higher access road but it will eventually be fully screened by fast growing trees.

The three lounges opening off the corridors are separated from the 'racetrack' corridors and are protected from through traffic, thereby affording a degree of intimacy and privacy. The small number of residents who may be disturbed, noisy and aggressive at any particular time use a small lounge on their own which enables the care staff to give them more personal attention.

In order to provide cues and clues for disoriented residents, each bedroom door contains a photograph of the occupant and their name printed in large lettering.

It is possible to open the front door from the outside but not from the inside so that no resident is at risk from wandering. This security is valued by the relatives of residents and is currently accepted as good practice consistent with the staff's duty to care under the common law. Management staff feel strongly that a lockable front door is far less restrictive and intrusive than various electronic and other security devices available. The interior courtyard and the secure external garden give a feeling of openness, lightness, spaciousness and freedom. A small private room adjacent to the front door is freely available for use by visitors, clergy, social workers or others who require an opportunity for private conversation.

A sense of intimacy is encouraged by the use of small tables in the dining room which also doubles as a function room. It contains a piano which is frequently played by visitors and some residents.

Bathrooms and toilets are spacious, well equipped and afford complete privacy although they are not lockable from the inside.

Extensive records are kept on each resident and are filed in the OIC's office. These contain a restricted section and the need for confidentiality is stressed with all staff and students. Confidentiality is specifically addressed on all in-service training programmes and in supervision sessions.

Review meetings are held in private in the OIC's office, a staff dining room is available for training events and a small visitors room is well used.

All residents are deemed incapable of managing their own affairs but the details of their financial circumstances are not held in Ferrard files but are known to the field social workers and the staff in the patients affairs office located at Holywell Hospital.

Information about the procedures followed in order to safeguard the property rights of residents is contained in the section on Rights. Only minimal financial information is held in the resident's personal file in Ferrard and it is contained in a restricted section of a comprehensive file.

This file is divided into separate sections covering the following:

- Residential application form, behaviour ratings and fieldwork report

- Progress charts and group assessments

- Progress reports and reviews

- Maintenance correspondence

- Medication and dental cards

- Professional and confidential letters

- Referral under Mental Health (Northern Ireland) Order 1986

- Harmful and damaging information

Many residents receive regular phone calls from relatives and they are always allowed to speak in private. Staff willingly assist anyone who wishes to make a phone call and they are then left to talk alone.

Without doubt the greatest single threat to privacy in Ferrard is the home's success. This results in a large number of professional visitors as well as social work students undertaking supervised practice placements. Great efforts are made to preserve privacy but it is not possible to prevent the presence of visitors impinging on the lives of residents. Visitors are introduced to residents whose surnames are always used in making introductions.

Staff are very aware of the need to safeguard privacy and confidentiality and to regard Ferrard as the home of the people who live in it. This is no easy task as its popularity constantly threatens its commitment to good practice in these matters and constant vigilance is needed to minimise intrusion.

DIGNITY

Recognition of the intrinsic value of people regardless of circumstances by respecting their uniqueness and their personal needs and treating them with respect.

The physical design of Ferrard which seeks to promote both privacy and dignity has already been described. The objectives of the home which are incorporated in a brochure include the objective 'to show sensitivity in coping with the dignity of the elderly person' and this principle is consistently addressed in staff training and supervision.

Each resident is invited to bring with them one piece of cherished furniture for their own bedroom. Otherwise furniture is standard although the colour schemes, curtains and bedspreads vary from room to room.

Residents are encouraged to have small ornaments and personal photographs and if someone does not have such ornaments these are provided. If any of these are broken or destroyed they are immediately replaced so that familiar surroundings are maintained and the person does not feel deprived or punished in any way. Flowers in the front hall and lounges are displayed all the year round and house plants abound.

A very high standard of personal hygiene and dress is maintained for all residents, especially the women who are helped by staff to take pride in their personal appearance. A hairdresser visits weekly and undertakes sets, trims and perms for residents and day care clients. Some residents who are accustomed to regular visits to the hairdresser continue to attend salons in the town.

Primary workers are responsible for bathing, keeping clothing in good order, assisting with its replacement and generally attending to the wellbeing of the residents for whom they have special responsibility. With staff encouragement most residents take considerable pride in their appearance. Everyone is well dressed and well groomed. Wearing shoes in the daytime is expected. Jewellery is worn, nails are kept short and well manicured and the everyday standard of personal dress and presentation is exceptionally high.

This pride in personal appearance is mirrored by management and care staff who do not wear uniform and who are expected to present themselves as participating in a job which requires high standards of personal care.

Bathing is undertaken by the primary worker with a flexibility which seeks to respect the wishes of the resident and to be consistent with their previous lifestyle in terms of preferred time of day, and frequency. It is always undertaken in complete privacy. A medic bath and a hoist have been augmented by the recent installation of a Parker bath which residents and staff find much more satisfactory. Showers are available but are less popular. Perhaps this is due to their relative unfamiliarity for people of this age.

Recreational therapy

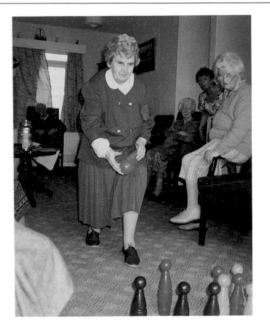

An active but sensitive continence management programme ensures the home is totally odour free. Without the programme all residents would be incontinent of urine and approximately one quarter, doubly incontinent. A small number who have not responded to retraining and regular toileting who continue to have faecal incontinence are managed on a special programme introduced and supervised by the psychogeriatrician. They are given daily codeine and a twice weekly enema which is administered by a visiting community nurse. This programme is justified in terms of a careful judgment which seeks to balance the indignity associated with repeated soiling and being cleaned up with the relative indignity of a twice weekly enema.

Staff are well pleased with the outcomes of this approach. Relatives are supportive and no resident has objected verbally or non verbally to the arrangements.

When a resident is first admitted, their toilet habits and routines are observed and recorded. Urinary incontinence is managed by a two hourly toileting regime. This usually re-establishes some degree of urinary control but also enhances personal well-being and means the home is free of

Wherever possible a resident's preference for the time of day for taking a bath is accommodated. By so doing their pleasure is enhanced and their compliance much more likely to be achieved. Relatives are encouraged to assist with the physical care of residents if they wish to do so. For some, this kind of involvement makes it easier for them to accept that they are no longer able to care for their relative within the community and to accept that they need to use the kind of sensitive help available in Ferrard.

smell. If a person is found to need more frequent toileting, a modified programme is introduced. Urinary tract infections are also readily identified because of the regular programme.

A similar approach is used with day care attenders. Many are bathed at Ferrard, thereby relieving anxious relatives of the responsibility for attending to the hygiene of people who are no longer able or interested, and are sometimes resistant in these matters.

Because of the continence programme, incontinence is not a problem. Therefore bathing does not assume the time consuming importance it occupies in many EMI homes. The appearance of the residents and the ethos of the home give no hint to the casual observer that a sophisticated programme of continence management is in operation.

Residents are usually addressed by their given names by care staff but invariably when spoken about at review meetings or handover meetings are called either Mr or Mrs X or by their combined given names and surnames.

Only if a resident's physical health seriously deteriorates and they go 'off their feet' will they be moved to the nearby hospital. Only rarely is it necessary to transfer a resident to the psychogeriatric unit of the local psychiatric hospital. Occasionally because of a severe functional illness or uncontrollable aggression which makes the person a risk to themselves and to others, will they be moved. With the steady growth in staff's competence and confidence, achieved through assiduous staff training over many years, exceedingly difficult behaviour can now be managed within Ferrard itself.

The close collaborative relationship with the psychogeriatrician based in Holywell Hospital, his ready accessibility and his detailed knowledge of all the residents means staff feel supported. They know that help, including if necessary a psychogeriatric bed, is readily available. Feeling supported they manage to cope with seriously disruptive and disturbed behaviour without needing to resort to the further indignity and confusion a hospital admission is liable to cause an already disturbed person.

INDEPENDENCE

Opportunities to act and think without reference to another person, including a willingness to incur a degree of calculated risk.

Wagner (1988) explained this principle as the need for residential staff to 'help and encourage residents to think and act independently as far as this is compatible with their own abilities, their impact on other people, the constraints of communal life, and the risks involved.' In an EMI home, the nature of the residents' impairment places some constraints on the degree of independence which can be extended to them.

Because of the risk of wandering, becoming lost and coming to harm, no resident is free to leave the unit unaccompanied. The front door is openable from the outside and locked on the inside.

All staff are trained and encouraged to be aware of the need to constantly find ways of maximising the independence of residents within this overall restriction of their freedom. The rationale for the most careful and detailed assessments, reviews and formulation of care plans is expressly for the purpose of helping residents maintain and retain, sometimes regain, whatever capacities they still have for independent action.

They are encouraged at all times to continue to undertake personal, social, recreational and cognitive tasks of which they are still capable. There is always an inherent tendency in institutions of all kinds to create what Seligman (1974) called 'learned dependency.' This tendency is a hazard of all residential homes and Ferrard is no exception to the insidious potential of perpetuating a staff-centred rather than a resident-centred regime. This inclination is only combated by vigilance, staff training and supervision and the courageous public commitment to alternative values.

Within the confines of the home, residents are free to use their bedrooms, move between sitting rooms and other areas, and participate or not in group activities. They may wander the corridors, although constructive occupation and diversion, together with careful monitoring of minimal medication reduces aimless wandering considerably.

They are allocated to a small group according to the detailed assessment of their needs and capabilities. This may be thought to be a curtailment of individual freedom and independence. In defence, the staff would energetically argue that Ferrard residents have genuine opportunities for continuing to be involved in meaningful pleasurable activity, unlike so many old people in residential care who spend their days as Godlove, Richard and Rodwell (1982) found, busy doing nothing.

Ferrard presents an active regime and the justification for its emphasis on group activities is persuasively supported by the evidence of happy busy people, so different from many conventional residential and nursing homes, and dramatically different from most EMI homes. The Ferrard programme supports the view of Burnside (1984) who argued so persuasively that

'The danger is not in the practice of group work with the elderly: the real danger is in not conducting groups and thereby fostering the still prevalent attitude of 'therapeutic nihilism'. It is better to take a risk than to sit by and watch apathy, fear, sensory deprivation, loneliness, and helplessness continue in the aged.'

The active involvement of relatives in a support group which is described in more detail elsewhere, is a powerful means by which the views of significant people who have a detailed knowledge of residents can be heeded. In effect it approximates to a consumer's view.

Independence is encouraged by residents going out to shop, to church, to visit relatives or on small planned outings. Most would leave Ferrard at least once a week. Many regularly visit relatives' homes for meals or overnight stays and join in family parties and celebrations.

No chemical or mechanical form of restraint is used, other than the lockable front door. There are no Buxton chairs or chairs with fixed tables attached. No mobility aids are permitted, neither zimmers nor walking sticks as they are considered a potential hazard to other residents. People who are not capable of walking unaided other than with the support provided by handrails along the walls of the corridors can not continue to live in Ferrard. If necessary they would have to be moved, not to the psychogeriatric ward of the local psychiatric hospital where similar rules about mobility aids apply, but to a ward in the local hospital, or very occasionally to a private nursing home.

Staff regret that because of policy and staffing provision they are unable to offer extended term terminal care. They feel their caring responsibilities are sometimes cut short as a consequence of the need to transfer a resident to hospital. If however a resident does fall seriously ill and has only a short time to live, they will be cared for at Ferrard. Following the death the body will be prepared before being moved by the undertaker. At the time admission is arranged the wishes of the nearest relative are always ascertained and recorded so that funeral arrangements may accord with the family's wishes.

Another factor which encourages independence in this environment is the availability of funds raised and controlled by the Relatives Support Group. This money is augmented by the judicious management of a devolved budget and staff and relatives work closely together to raise money. The support group has contributed many of the additional homely touches which facilitate freedom and independence. Of recent years they have bought a microwave oven, additional furniture, a reality orientation board for the dining room, and contributed to the costs of developing the reminiscence garden. Free monies encourage a free spirit and both are apparent in Ferrard.

CHOICE

The opportunity to select from a range of options.

Many of the issues concerning choice have already been covered in the sections on privacy, dignity and independence. As with all these quality of life indicators, it is inappropriate to discuss them in absolutist terms or without reference to the context in which people live and work.

To extend genuine choice to people with dementia in residential and day care services requires tremendous vigilance and an open willingness to scrutinise one's own practice. Staff from both the Unit of Management and Ferrard work hard to make a range of realistic choices possible for recipients of the dementia service.

Choice depends on the availability of alternatives. In the Ferrard model of care, the alternatives are more numerous, accessible, flexible, acceptable and effective than in many, and probably most dementia services.

Through the provision of the various services like early assessment, domiciliary support, laundry, respite and day care, there is a real choice about whether to enter residential care or to continue to live in the community.

It is wrong to infer that prior to admission people had free choice and that after admission, choice is renounced or much curtailed. For some people, their dementing illness has long since curtailed the quality of life for themselves and their relatives, and by admission to care wider choice becomes possible. For most, the relative loss of their independence and curtailment of free choice have to be traded off against gains in personal security, enhanced social care and stimulation which group living offers.

People who after careful assessment become permanent residents in Ferrard are cared for by staff who seek to understand their past history, personal preferences, and their likes and dislikes. This extensive knowledge is then used to maintain as much of the familiar as possible and to sensitively establish residents in a new environment with new patterns of living.

Allocation to a care group within the home is made on the basis of detailed assessment which is described elsewhere. Once allocated to a care group and to a primary worker, staff try hard to extend

choice, within limited options, in many small but none the less significant ways.

Because the assessment is so detailed and the knowledge of past history reasonably extensive, staff are able to make decisions, where the degree of impairment prevents the person doing so, more in terms of the principle of 'substituted judgment' and less in terms of the conventional 'best interests' test so commonly used by professional carers. In the light of knowledge about past life style, interests and occupation, they try to decide, as best they can, what

Craft-work

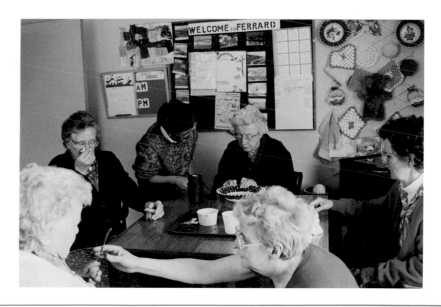

the resident would have chosen for herself had she been able to do so. In substantial areas of daily living, however, residents are well able to exercise their own judgment and make their own choices and they are given every opportunity to do so.

To claim that this is always done and that staff never make quick expedient decisions which serve the routines and needs of the institution rather than the needs of the individual would be unrealistic. It is claimed however that Ferrard staff seem more aware than many, and more able than most, to express an awareness of the issues and to demonstrate appropriate and self-conscious discipline.

Whether or not rooms have to be shared mostly depends on availability. As the occupancy level is virtually a hundred per cent choice in this matter is very limited, especially when every effort is made to give restless wandering people with disturbed sleep patterns a single room in order to minimise disturbance to others. Unless a resident clearly indicates they wish to continue sharing they will be transferred to a single room as soon as one becomes available.

CLOTHING

All residents receive new clothing at least twice yearly. Whenever possible, primary workers, relatives or both take residents on individual shopping trips in the local town. They travel by taxi and tend to shop in places where through long association, the retail staff is well known for their sensitivity and patience. One shop brings clothing to Ferrard twice a year so in this way choice can be broadened and extended with residents having the opportunity to shop in leisurely privacy.

Variety and quality are apparent in the clothing worn which is all individually marked and laundered on the premises. It is paid for from personal allowances which are banked weekly on behalf of each resident and managed by the staff responsible for patients' affairs at Holywell hospital.

Genuine free choice is exercised over many aspects of daily living. For example the time of day when a resident is known to be less confused will be used by a key worker to get them to select their own clothes to wear the following day, take a bath or read them a letter.

MEALS

The significance of food and mealtimes is clearly recognised by both domestic and care staff. Individual choice about mealtimes is balanced with the need to provide a structure and order to the resident's day which helps them retain their contact with the here and now. The tension and inherent contradiction between a simultaneous commitment to 'freedom' and 'patterning' is very relevant to the management of meals and mealtimes.

Some choice is permitted over the time of getting up and going to bed but great care is taken to adhere to life long patterns. Most residents are early risers but one woman who all her life never got up before 10.00am still lies on and then makes her own breakfast with minimal help in the day care bungalow. Thus her life long habits are respected and her self care skills preserved.

An unhurried approach to mealtimes is very apparent and two sittings are used to accommodate residents and day care attenders. Round wooden tables seat three or four people. Food is served by care staff through a large open hatchway to the kitchen. The cook is an integral part of the caring team and is thoroughly committed to the Ferrard way of life. Her statement 'I know everyone and keep my eyes open' is borne out by her specific attention to the needs of individuals.

Residents' past preferences and food habits help determine the menu which is varied from day to day. The main meal is served in the middle of the day between 12.00–1.00pm and consists of a main course and pudding. Breakfast is available from 8.30–9.30am and tea from 4.00–5.00pm. Supper is served between 7.30–8.30pm or later depending on evening entertainment and drinks are available mid morning and mid afternoon or anytime on request. Popular Ulster food such as potato bread, soda farls and wheaten bread is regularly served.

If someone has been a vegetarian prior to admission or to have other dietary preferences with a religious or ethnic basis these are always respected.

A relatively high carbohydrate diet is offered, partly because of its familiarity and partly because people who are restless or agitated require higher food intakes than people who are more sedentary. Body weight is carefully monitored by monthly weighing.

Housework

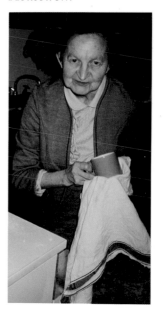

In keeping with the life experience of most residents a roast is only served on Sundays in order to enhance peoples' ability to locate themselves in time and continue familiar patterns of life.

Birthdays are always celebrated individually and a special cake provided.

The first sitting for meals includes everyone who can feed themselves without assistance and those who enjoy being involved in some of the domestic chores associated with setting and clearing tables. One resident regards herself as 'on the staff' and she has significant responsibilities in the dining room.

Some others who appreciate the individual freedom of managing their own arrangements sit at tables set with milk jugs, sugar bowls and small tea pots. For others, beverages are poured and sugar added by staff to help residents preserve socially acceptable eating habits.

Fluid intake is carefully monitored for everyone and great trouble is taken to coax reluctant people to drink.

People who are either very slow eaters or who are unable to feed themselves attend the second sitting and are assisted by staff and some residents who like to help. This is an unhurried process and people are lovingly encouraged to eat at their own pace.

Smokers are provided with cigarettes by staff at the end of each meal. They sit on, leisurely smoking, sometimes talking to each other or to staff, and generally behaving as if they were in their own homes.

If people lose their appetite they will be tempted by small helpings of specially prepared food, now made much easier because of a microwave oven purchased by the support group. It is also used to prepare suppertime drinks where the choice covers tea, coffee, horlicks, cocoa and milk. The microwave also makes it possible to quickly respond to the needs of a restless or sleepless resident.

Originally Ferrard had a cook but the post was relinquished to save money to fund the domiciliary care worker's post. At this time meals were supplied ready cooked by the hospital kitchen. In the recent past catering services have been privatised throughout the Unit of Management and Ferrard has reinstated the positions of cook and assistant cook because of the conviction that responsive accessible catering is a cornerstone of the type of caring ethos Ferrard is determined to preserve.

The interior courtyard and the new external garden provide choice within safe boundaries. As so many residents come from rural backgrounds, staff are working to lessen the 'town' feel of the house and garden and to devise, design and incorporate more familiar country features.

Small group outings to familiar places and favourite haunts are common. Television is used sparingly, not as background noise. Residents are read short poems and stories, often in local dialect. They are encouraged to sing favourite songs and listen to familiar music. Old tunes, not modern pop are played for dancing, movement and exercise sessions.

Key workers help residents remember and celebrate significant events such as an anniversary or a relative's birthday and to continue to be involved in family activities albeit often in more limited ways.

Residents are encouraged to join in family outings, visit friends and relations for occasional meals and go away for holidays.

If family outings are not possible, a key worker will arrange outings for either an individual or a small group. Large outings, especially in buses are considered inappropriate.

MEDICAL CARE

Residents do not retain their own general practitioners. On permanent admission they join the list of a doctor in the local group practice situated nearby. Everyone is routinely screened for vision and hearing problems on admission.

A closed loop system is fitted in one lounge to assist residents who have hearing difficulties.

It is frequently possible to reduce medication after admission especially the use of sedatives and tranquillisers. All drugs are carefully monitored with the general practitioner and psychogeriatrician working very closely together. A Kardex system is used for controlling drugs and their reordering is the responsibility of the night senior care assistant.

All residents are medically assessed as being incapable of managing their own

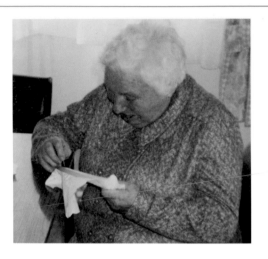

affairs and accordingly they are no longer entitled to vote in local or national elections.

In summary it can be said that these people whose mental state has resulted in the need for them to reside in an EMI home experience significant limitations to the exercise of unfettered free choice. Nevertheless, within the limitations identified, every effort is made within Ferrard to maximise the opportunities for exercising circumscribed choice.

RIGHTS

The maintenance of all entitlements associated with citizenship

With the implementation of 'People First' (1990) statutory residential facilities in Northern Ireland are in the process of becoming subject to exactly the same monitoring arrangements by arms length inspection units as pertain in the voluntary and private sectors. Eventually it is intended that day care provision will also be subjected to similar arrangements.

In the past the Line Manager has been responsible for ensuring standards, initiating planning, making initial investigations of complaints at the same time as being closely involved in admission and review panels and in supervising the head of home and participating in staff training. The disentangling of monitoring, inspection and complaints investigation from managerial responsibility for the quality of care is welcomed as it should provide greater protection for vulnerable people.

At present the general standards of residential care in the Northern Health and Social Services Board appear to be enhanced within Ferrard. This is explained by a number of different but interdependent factors such as clarity about the philosophy of care, agreed operational objectives, high expectations, active staff induction and on-going training, considerable participation by various professions and the active involvement of residents' families and friends.

Within the general commitment to safeguarding rights, the day to day programme of care emphasises respect, courtesy, privacy, especially in matters concerned with bathing and toileting, careful attention to personal grooming and a sensitivity to individual differences.

Ferrard is entirely free from any smell of urine, no small achievement when all residents would be singly incontinent, and a substantial number, doubly incontinent, were it not for the active continence management programme.

This programme is based on the careful recording of each resident's behaviour and the systematic consistent implementation of a programme which usually consists of two hour toileting.

The physical environment has been rendered as safe as possible in inconspicuous ways which have not sacrificed homeliness or comfort. Pictures are unobtrusively secured to the walls, furniture is carefully chosen, sitting rooms are softened with wool carpets and the corridors are fitted with handrails.

The risks attendant on wandering are eliminated by securing the front door which is considered a less obtrusive safety measure than either pressure mats or electronic tagging.

Property rights are safeguarded by referral to the Master of Care and Protection who is responsible for the management of the estates of people who are deemed incapable. The residential staff are not involved in financial matters other than pensions and personal allowances. Field social workers at the time of admission determine whether or not enduring power of attorney exists. If not, once a person is medically judged to be incapable they are referred to the Master who will either appoint a committee or the public solicitor to act on person's behalf.

The Head of Unit is the receiving officer for the receipt of pensions. All residents contribute according to their means and the weekly rate varies from £41.60 to £217.00. Everyone receives a personal allowance of £10.40 but this is not handled by the residents who only ever have minimal small change available to them. The personal allowances are banked with the office of patients' affairs in Holywell Hospital and used for purchasing clothing, outings and holidays.

The right to practice their religion is respected. It is worth noting that sectarian bitterness which bedevils so much of Ulster life has never been an issue for either residents or staff in Ferrard where people live and work together without bitterness or dissension. Reflecting the demography of the catchment area, there are more Protestant than Catholic residents and fair employment practices are monitored by the Northern Health and Social Services Board.

Stitching

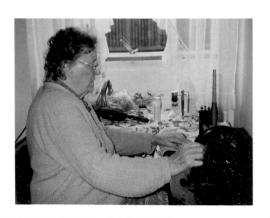

Local Protestant clergy take it in turns to hold a weekly afternoon inter-denominational service which is held in the dining room. To provide continuity each minister takes four consecutive services. The service consists of short readings, prayers, familiar hymns and a short address. Sometimes a resident plays the piano and sometimes the visiting minister is accompanied by the church organist.

Residents are reminded that the service is being held and they are free to attend or not as they choose.

Some residents are taken to church services in the town on Sunday mornings, travelling by taxi and accompanied by a care assistant. Others watch services on television.

The Roman Catholic priest conducts a monthly service in the home and residents frequently attend mass in the local chapel.

Anyone who requests a visit from their priest or clergyman will have the request conveyed straight away.

To some limited extent residents are free to choose their daily companions but in so far as they are allocated to small groups on the basis of assessments made by staff, they are less free to choose their own company than they might otherwise be if no small group activities were available.

Where residents have known each other prior to admission, have come from the same locality or have expressed any friendship preferences, they are encouraged by staff to spend time together, to sit together in the dining room or to share other activities.

The maintenance of responsibility for self, notwithstanding cognitive impairment, is paramount. This means in practice that key workers conscientiously seek to enhance personal choice in every way possible and so respect the rights of each individual within a group context. The task of balancing an individual's rights and the rights of all other individuals within the residential home is complex and calls for constant vigilance on the part of all concerned. Ferrard staff are aware of the problems and they struggle honestly with the dilemmas posed by their residents who are vulnerable people living private lives in public places.

Maslow (1954) suggested a hierarchy of human needs. Attention to physiological needs, safety, love and belonging, esteem, achievement and recognition, self-actualisation and the desire to know and to understand are all addressed in Ferrard House.

As in most residential homes, physiological and safety needs are well taken care of. The other more intangible needs are more difficult to attend to in any institutional setting. They are particularly difficult to address consistently in an institution for people whose cognitive deficits put them at daily risk of being dismissed as non-people.

Ferrard seeks to create an environment which is the very antithesis of Miller and Gwynne's (1974) 'warehousing' model. Rather it seeks to create and sustain a 'horticultural' model in which people's needs for love and belonging are addressed both by staff and relatives.

FULFILMENT

The realisation of personal aspirations and abilities in all aspects of daily life.

People's achievements are acknowledged, and their past valued so that they can be genuinely esteemed. The key worker system fosters the possibility for close warm relationships to gradually evolve. People are appreciated for their own sakes. The things they can still do rather than not do are stressed. Loss and sadness are not denied but life in Ferrard is for living to the full as far as that is possible, notwithstanding personal pain and present limitations.

Self actualisation is almost impossible to assess in people who are unable to give an account of themselves yet in many small ways hints of pleasure, happiness and satisfaction can be inferred from observed behaviour. Skilled sensitive staff find time to share in the lives of residents in many small ways despite the burden of physical care tasks. There is time to sit and chat, to share a joke, read a newspaper or a letter, or to take trouble over some particularly personal matter.

Ferrard residents are alive and lively. They are neither busy doing nothing nor heavily sedated. Medication is used sparingly and challenging behaviour, which certainly exists, is managed by increased personal attention, distraction and diversion.

Except for mobility aids which put other people at risk, all other aids and adaptations which could assist anyone maintain independence are used. Because walking aids and walking sticks are prohibited, this may mean that a resident whose mobility deteriorates but who is otherwise happy and well settled may have to be transferred for the good of the greater number. Such a resident's opportunities for fulfilment may have to be sacrificed in the interests of others.

Grouping residents in terms of their ability, compatibility and behaviour, a special kind of adult streaming, is the most effective means so far devised by management staff to reconcile individual and group needs. The quietly conforming undemanding resident is guaranteed attention by her key worker although there is no doubt that the noisy, aggressive, hyperactive people demand, and receive more attention, especially attention from senior staff.

The sexual needs of residents are only implicitly understood. This subject is receiving increasing attention and is likely to be included in future staff training because concern is growing about the number of cases of suspected elder abuse and exploitation, some with sexual connotations which are coming to notice.

IN-HOUSE GROUPWORK

Once a person has been assessed either by having a short term admission or through attendance at the day centre and it has been agreed they should become a resident, then a detailed care plan is drawn up. They are allocated to a key worker for the purpose of personal care and to a small group for the purpose of daily occupation and social stimulation.

Small groups are held in the various sitting rooms and living areas of Ferrard and are led by care assistants with the clear recognition that this work is an integral part of their job and their other caring tasks are arranged to make this possible.

The programme for the in-house groups is planned a week in advance by the senior care staff. Its content is determined by the interests and skills of the care staff available and the needs of the residents. Groups are held both mornings and afternoons. Evenings, other than Wednesday night's Friendship Club are less structured but often informal entertainment

and small group activities are organised by staff and visitors.

These groups seek to provide interesting activities within the scope of each resident's capacities, interest and attention span. The daily groupwork programme challenges the 'unknowability' of dementia. It guarantees that staff notice residents who are both audible and visible. They are treated as real people who are given serious sensitive attention both as individuals and as members of small groups.

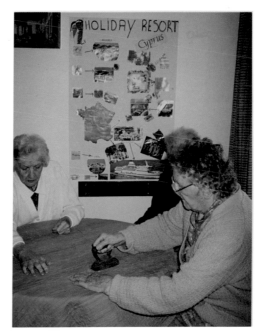

Ironing

45

The outline programme for a week is given in Appendix 4 . Reminiscence, personal care, music and movement, simple crafts and conversation are all encouraged. Staff have grown very skilled in improvising equipment and making the most of the spontaneous as well as the planned opportunities for constructive occupation and socialisation which abound when the established ethos encourages positive rather than negative attitudes towards people's capabilities.

Individual wishes about participating in any of the small groups are respected. If a person indicates either by verbal or non verbal means they do not wish to participate and prefers to be alone or uninvolved in any activity they are not pressed into a programme.

The care staff by means of in-service training and opportunities to attend short courses and conferences, are helped to develop groupwork skills and to acquire skills associated with specific activities or therapeutic approaches.

The natural flair, aptitudes and experience of the care staff are fully utilised in this work which seeks to ensure that the cognitive capacities which people retain are stimulated and used, and that they have enjoyable occupation which is usually undertaken in the company of other people. The emphasis is on using peoples strengths not emphasising their deficits.

Very restless or agitated residents and anyone with aggressive and challenging behaviour are managed in a very small group, usually with no more than three or four members. Some residents participate in the more intensive and tightly structured day care programme in the bungalow for some days each week.

There is an ever present tendency in most caring relationships, formal or informal, to restrict choice, to do things for the impaired person rather than to let them take the time to do things for themselves, and thus to accelerate their dependency. Carers act in this way through good intention rather than malevolence. Constant management oversight is needed in Ferrard as elsewhere to minimise this inherent tendency in highly motivated caring staff. It is a seeming contradiction at the very heart of their work and one which receives major attention in staff training and supervision.

FRIENDSHIP CLUB

This Club meets every Wednesday evening in the dining room at Ferrard. Four voluntary entertainers take it in turns to provide a programme of live music, singing, dancing and other recreation.

The purpose is entirely social although the therapeutic spin-off from shared good fun, social stimulation and contact with other people should not be minimised.

People living either on their own in the community or with relatives are free to attend and again this increases their familiarity with Ferrard. They are not intrusive as their numbers are small and they are made to feel very welcome by the staff.

This club is proof that conscientious volunteers who are prepared to make a regular commitment can be recruited and that their contribution enriches and extends the resources available to the residential care staff. This kind of community involvement has to be cultivated and nurtured. It rarely happens without effort but Ferrard has proved that the rewards can be considerable.

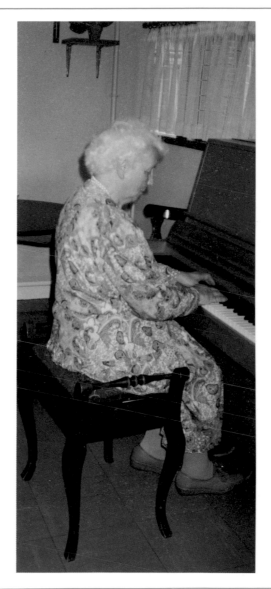

Music therapy

6

DAY CARE

The small bungalow adjoining the main house which is no longer required for staff accommodation is being effectively used as a small intimate day centre. It has direct access as well as being immediately accessible to the main house and the new garden. It consists of a larger room, smaller room, kitchen and lavatory. Another small room provides an office for the domiciliary care worker and enables her to keep in close contact with the day care worker.

The large room is comfortably furnished with tables and chairs and is used as the major activities room. Eight to ten people can use the room at a time. The domestic scale of the building helps promote the programme so much of which is aimed at preserving basic social, personal and domestic skills and helping people who have lost such skills regain some competence.

The smaller room is furnished and equipped as a reminiscence room which has an impressive collection of local artefacts, memorabilia and other multi-sensory reminiscence trigger materials.

This building and the programme offered within it provides some Ferrard residents with a change from the main house. It offers involvement in specific programmes for carefully defined objectives, including assessment of both residents and people living in the community. Respite for family carers is an important part of this work.

The policy statement for the day care programme states:

Aim: To provide a more supportive environment for the client which will focus primarily upon maximising the independence and social adaptation of the individual and family unit.

Objectives:

1 To carry out a detailed assessment on each client and formulate a care plan.

2 To assist in the development of self confidence and self awareness through groupwork and counselling.

3 To assist clients to relearn basic skills, including social, domestic and community living skills.

4 To support and educate the immediate carers in the management of problems with activities of daily living.

There are clearly defined criteria for admission to the day care programme which apply equally to Ferrard residents and to people still living in the community.

They are as follows:

1 Clients must be fully ambulant.

2 Clients must not be doubly incontinent.

3 It must be established that the needs of the individual can not be met by any other means such as an old people's club or voluntary organisation.

4 The day care staff must be able to formulate and implement an appropriate programme of social care.

5 All clients are admitted initially for a four week assessment period.

6 The number of days on which a person attends is decided in consultation with either the residential primary and key workers and the domiciliary care worker.

The application form used is given in Appendix 5.

Staffing is provided by one full-time member of the senior care staff who is assisted from time to time by other care staff.

The small group activities are varied and imaginative. Great attention is paid to group process and activities are used as a means to enhance sociability, preserve skills and give pleasure in achievement. From the programme included as Appendix (6) the framework for a week can be seen. The activities include reality orientation, craft work, sewing, knitting, story telling, poetry reading, painting, modelling, reminiscence, music and cooking. As with the in-house groups, the work is carefully planned but it is never so rigid that opportunities for spontaneous developments, conversation and activities are lost. The programme is simultaneously planned and flexible, both essential characteristics if the needs of the client group are to be effectively addressed. Whilst many activities are task focused because a tangible achievement builds confidence, product and process are equally important.

A lot of project work is built around the seasons, special festivals, events and celebrations. For example in the last year people have knitted blankets for a third world relief project, celebrated the Queen Mother's ninetieth birthday, won a prize with a collage in an Age Concern craft competition, drawn and painted pictures on themes of Guy Fawkes and Halloween, and made Christmas cards. Many successful small group activities are undertaken in which each person makes a contribution according to their level of interest, capacity and concentration. Tasks are broken down into small components and the worker's job is to plan, encourage, guide, teach and co-ordinate. Cooking and other domestic tasks are well suited

to this co-operative approach.

For example in a sandwich-making session up to six people are involved in different aspects of the activity. Two butter the bread, one grates cheese, another mashes corn beef, mixing in sauce with two others spreading the fillings on the bread. The prepared sandwiches are then eaten for afternoon tea, a sociable event in which everyone participates and the washing up is undertaken, usually very competently, by a couple of the members.

The day care programme is closely integrated into the rest of Ferrard and its ongoing small group care work. It is an integral part of the whole, not a separate or competitive enterprise. Because of this it is easy for a restless member who may fail to settle in the relatively close confines of the bungalow on any particular day, to return to the main house. Here they may get involved in an alternative group activity or be free to wander the corridors if physical exercise better meets their needs of the moment.

The programme is not rigidly adhered to so that extra mural activities may be easily incorporated. A small number of people going for an outing by car, a birthday celebration, attendance at the local Silver Threads Club in the town, or some other event, either spontaneous or planned can readily be fitted into the programme.

Over the years close links have been painstakingly developed with local voluntary organisations whose contributions to Ferrard and its residents are highly valued. Local churches and youth groups, St. Vincent de Paul Society, Legion of Mary, Women's Institute and the British Legion make regular visits throughout the whole year. Lately members of a local Mothers' Union Group have begun to offer a sitting service to enable carers to attend the Relatives' Support Group.

This community involvement means that staff feel supported, not isolated, residents have wider involvements than many in similar homes and relatives know that other people understand something about the nature of dementia.

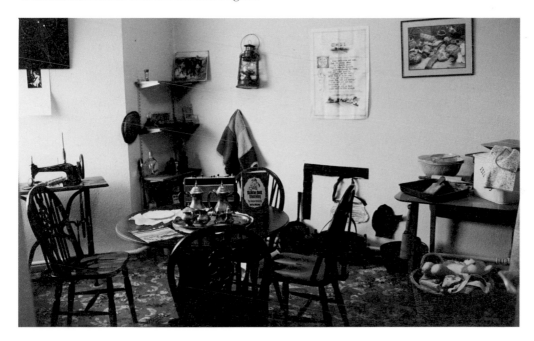

Reminiscence room

Day care linked to a period in residence, or managed from the community has assessment and rehabilitative objectives for many people. It is used to either extend the possibility of the person continuing to live in the community in a domestic setting or becoming able to live in an alternative community setting such as a conventional residential home.

The rehabilitation programme seeks to identify potential clients, introduce them to the service, plan, monitor and record a programme of care. Very specific goals are set and progress towards each is evaluated through careful observation and meticulous daily recording and written weekly summaries.

Families are fully involved in this process. If it is agreed that the person with dementia should be placed in an alternative residential setting, they and clients are sensitively introduced to any new residential setting which is proposed. Initially short visits are made to familiarise the person with the new location and the times of visits are gradually extended.

Once a placement has been made, the Ferrard staff will slowly decrease contact over a four to six week period when contact will cease and a discharge from the Ferrard service is recorded.

In the last five years 14 residents who participated in the Ferrard rehabilitation programme have been placed successfully in alternative conventional residential care and four, supported by various means, have returned to live in their own homes. It is not possible to say how many non-residents have been maintained in the community and for how long but impressionistic evidence supports the claim that this relatively small inexpensive type of programme is very cost effective.

7

DOMICILIARY OUTREACH SERVICE

The domiciliary outreach work gradually evolved from the residential and day care developments. At first when a carer known to Ferrard needed assistance with a relative living in the community, whatever senior member of the Ferrard staff who could be spared would visit them at home. This service was difficult to staff, lacked continuity and was not conducive to the establishment of high quality practice. It quickly became apparent that if this service was to fulfil its potential a specific worker was required. Initially the funding was found within the Ferrard staff budget by relinquishing domestic staff and using the hospital catering service. The position was established at the level of one senior care assistant working 20 hours a week and having an essential car user's allowance. Funding has since been secured with contributions from fieldwork services as well as residential care budgets.

To describe the outreach work separately is to distort its complete integration into the rest of the Ferrard programme. It is a crucial dimension and serves as a bridge between in-house and extra mural aspects of the dementia service.

From the time the post was established as a separate permanent job, continuity and stability have been provided as it has been held by the same person. The domiciliary worker may accept referrals from any source but most originate either with the field social workers or the psychogeriatrician.

The service is designed to help maintain people in the community for as long as possible and if it becomes necessary, smooth their transition into residential care. This is achieved either by direct support if the person lives alone or through the training, support and relief of carers.

Those who live alone and those who live with others are facilitated in gaining access to a range of residential, day care and other resources. The service is a tangible demonstration of the philosophy of shared care.

The worker is managerially responsible to the Community Manager (Dementia Service) and is supervised by her. She has considerable freedom and flexibility in her use of time. Her case load consists of approximately 40 people who live in the Antrim/Ballymena catchment area.

Working closely with two field social workers attached to teams in the Antrim and Ballymena fieldwork offices, the domiciliary worker supports carers, maintains existing networks, and offers information and advice about day to day management of difficult behaviour. She acts as a well sign-posted pathway for people both into and out of Ferrard House and its associated day care facility.

The service is characterised by:
- open referral
- ready availability
- flexibility
- creative imagination
- responsiveness

The domiciliary worker makes early contact with any new referral and in this way establishes herself as a known, familiar and trusted source of advice and information. She explains as often as necessary what services are available. She assists in arranging short term admissions for assessment and respite, she reacts sensitively to carer's changing needs as the condition of the person with dementia alters, and she helps to plan and co-ordinate an appropriate response.

She is there, not to obstruct access to the service but rather to facilitate, not to create barriers but to make it possible for people to use the help which is available. She is there, not to create dependency but to sustain carers for as long as they wish and are able to care.

It is recognised that many carers find it difficult to share care for a variety of complex reasons. Their present caring demands must be seen within the context of the history of past relationships and understood in terms of the carer's expectations which they hold of themselves and other family members. Counselling carers is a skilled task and no one professional in the Ferrard service has a monopoly. It is shared by various people but falls most heavily on the field social worker and the domiciliary care worker.

The service which the latter offers is a mix of practical advice, direct service, and warm caring support. Carers are often helped to plan a weekly programme of stimulation and activity. Careful detailed training about managing aberrant behaviours is given and often carers are encouraged to compile and use a life history photograph album or a life story book, techniques which have proved to be very rewarding with some people. Help can be given to transport people to either Ferrard or another nearer residential home for bathing, lunch or a social event. Carers are encouraged to attend the Carers' Support Group which is less fearsome when they know the domiciliary worker will be present.

She is a trusted familiar participant in the Support Group. Along with other senior staff she plays an important role in encouraging relatives to express their needs, their feelings and the conflicts as well as the satisfactions inherent in caring.

Use of the incontinence laundry service is expedited by the domiciliary worker as well as access to daycare, the lunch club and informal occasional day or night sitting and respite care.

Since the recent extension of the geographic area covered by the Unit of Management a second domiciliary care worker has been appointed in order to provide a similar service to people living in these rural and urban areas. Until a second residential facility has been developed, people requiring respite care will be accommodated in Ferrard House and the domiciliary worker will do everything possible to help families make effective use of this resource.

Needle-craft

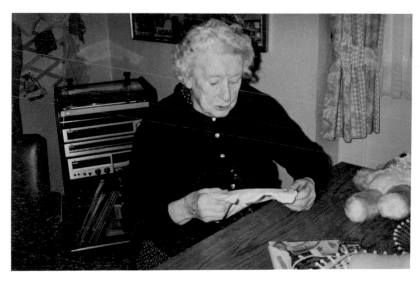

A 'panic button' service is also available though actually is seldom used. Carers are able to telephone Ferrard any time of the day or night if they are faced with difficult behaviour they are unable to manage. Ferrard notifies the OIC and contacts the domiciliary worker who visits immediately. She is able to offer whatever help is appropriate and support the relative in their distress.

The worker is rarely called out but the existence of the service provides security and reassurance to the carers. It engenders a conviction they are not struggling isolated and alone, that someone cares for them in their predicament and that should they need it, help is at hand.

Art therapy

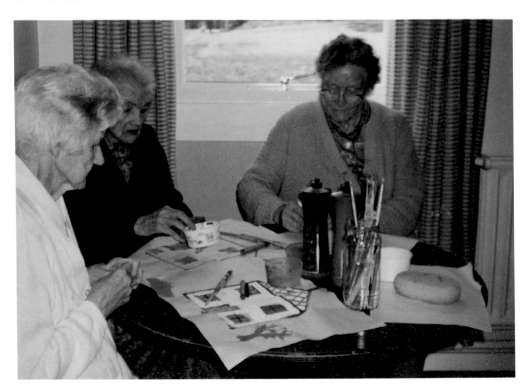

The domiciliary worker's role overlaps with the responsibilities of several other members of the dementia care team. The field social worker is responsible for compiling a detailed life and developmental history as well as gathering information about present social and financial circumstances. The domiciliary care worker and the day care worker are responsible for assessments of current functional competence. The general practitioner and the psychogeriatrician assess physical, emotional and cognitive capacities. If the person is admitted to Ferrard for assessment, residential staff will contribute their observations and experience which will cover the whole 24 hour cycle. It is likely that community psychiatric nurses will become more involved in the dementia service in the future and their contribution will need to be clarified. Working in a multi-disciplinary team characterised by cooperative collaborative work, the information will be pooled, decisions made and responsibility for the implementation of action plans agreed.

INTER-DISCIPLINARY WORKING RELATIONSHIPS

This is an important practical service which helps sustain people living either alone or with relatives in the community. It is a small service in terms of the numbers served, 12 people in 1990–91 who had some 5,264 items of a personal and household nature laundered. Currently seven people are receiving this service, which is highly valued by carers. Its marginal costs are small because it is run as an adjunct to the existing laundry work undertaken in Ferrard but its benefits are considerable in terms of sustaining people in the community. The concept 'shared care' rather than 'respite care' more accurately reflects the Ferrard approach. Respite is but one aspect of a multi-faceted service where carers, paid and unpaid, formal and informal, share together the complex demanding task of sustaining people with dementia.

INCONTINENCE LAUNDRY SERVICE

8

SHARED OR RESPITE CARE

Short term care has long been a part of the continuum of care based on Ferrard. It has gradually evolved over time, growing in flexibility and sophistication. To ensure its availability one bed is now designated specifically for respite and/or assessment. The service is characterised by imaginative flexibility and carers are helped to make effective use of a service characterised by the concepts of shared care and partnership in care.

Some families like to plan regular breaks while others prefer to use the service occasionally on an ad hoc basis to cover family exigencies or special events. Others may not have used the service at all but regard its existence as a reassurance knowing that if at some future time their own capacity to care is eroded, relief will be available.

For some older people and their carers it is a stepping stone towards the day when deterioration makes permanent residential care necessary.

The extent of participation in shared care which may be either on a short term residential basis or day attendance is determined by need. Evening and weekend care is also available either regularly or to enable a carer to attend a special event. Attendance at the Wednesday evening Friendship Club is also encouraged.

LUNCH CLUB

To increase familiarity with Ferrard and relieve carers, a small number of people come to Ferrard for lunch and to participate if they want to in any afternoon activities. Staff are aware of the risks inherent in using a residential facility as a community resource as discussed by Allen (1986). Because the numbers attending at any one time are small they are readily absorbed into the ongoing life of Ferrard and do not seem to detract from the quality of life of the permanent residents.

Day attenders may also be bathed or have their hair done. Some carers find these tasks extremely difficult to achieve at home so by offering this help family stress is often reduced or eliminated and carers are enabled to continue caring.

If a relative finds it difficult to get the person with dementia to co-operate in attending dental, optical, chiropody or hospital appointments, the domiciliary care worker or another member of the Ferrard staff is able to accompany them. They assist in ways which seek to increase the skills and confidence of the carer, not to undermine them. Similar help is offered to people who are living alone in the community who may be too forgetful or too disorganised to keep appointments.

Short term admissions may primarily be for respite but they often also fulfil an assessment function. Some are arranged specifically to enable a detailed assessment to be undertaken. Admission for the lat-

ter purpose is common but not routine. Its use is always carefully weighed up because it is often more informative to see someone functioning in their own familiar environment without subjecting them to the likelihood of increased disorientation when they are removed to unfamiliar surroundings.

From long experience staff are convinced that people who have had the admission process carefully attended to, and who are not rushed or hijacked into residential care are much more likely to settle with minimal distress. Proper attention to admission leads to more successful transition and eventual incorporation into the daily life of the residential home.

Everyone who is undergoing assessment either on a residential or day basis participates in the structured day care programme in the day centre. Following a period of assessment a care plan will be drawn up. Some people will continue to attend for day relief and some for a more structured programme with specific objectives which may include training, and rehabilitation, socialisation, occupation and carer relief.

For several years a support group has met one evening a month in the day centre bungalow. Initially it included only the relatives of residents but as the services based on Ferrard have been extended so the group has expanded to embrace carers of people with dementia who are living in the community.

The group seeks to provide a friendly sociable meeting place for people facing a common problem and attendance varies from 6–20 with an average of approximately 10. It offers people mutual support, encouragement, information and advice and an opportunity to contribute in practical ways to the development of services for people with dementia. It provides a safe place for carers to talk about their struggles and to face their own limitations.

The domiciliary worker attends and other senior staff including the day care worker take it in turns to participate. The leadership of the group is very firmly in the hands of its members who are warmly welcoming, articulate and secure in their relationships with staff. As in many mutual aid support groups there is a tension between those members who wish to use the meetings to work on their own feelings such as anger, frustration, sadness, depression, guilt, and self criticism over their shortcomings as carers and those who wish to contribute through organising functions and by fund raising.

Despite the tensions over objectives there is a high degree of mutual concern and respect amongst members. Some long established participants are extremely supportive of newcomers and skilled in encouraging them to voice their pain in addition to mobilising their talents and involving them in money raising projects.

The Group is very clear about only using the money it raises for the direct benefit of the residents and others with dementia. For example recent purchases have included a microwave oven and a reality orientation board for the dining room so helping extend choice and improve and enrich the care environment.

Fund raising has enabled the Group to contribute towards the cost of the new reminiscence garden and members will be much involved in its official opening and in using it as a venue for future garden parties and other money raising functions.

Ability and willingness to raise money obviously makes the relatives a valued asset to the staff as well as to the residents. Carers however are recognised as having needs in their own right. Each one's reaction to the caring experience is different and their unique response is acknowledged. They too are respected and their needs addressed. The mutual aid function of the Group is clearly recognised as an important dimension. Staff share with established members the roles of facilitators and enablers in this process.

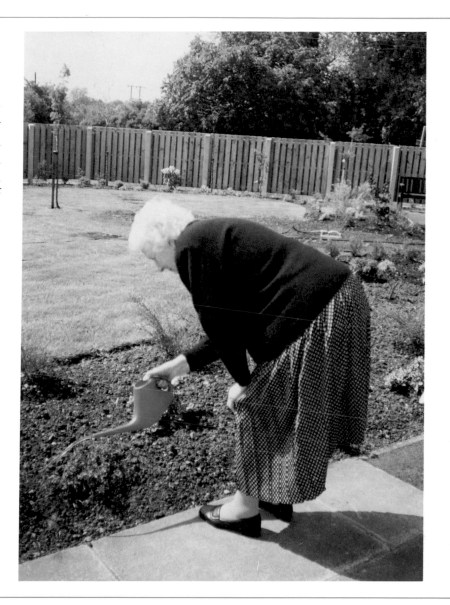

Gardening

9

CONCLUSION

As Ferrard House and the community dementia services which have grown from it face the future two separate tensions are apparent. The new climate created by the philosophy espoused in *People First* which is driven by managerial accountability and has spawned the new world of contracting and value for money in a mixed economy of care is one such tension. The other is an equally strong emphasis on quality assurance, consumerism and attention to the needs of carers.

The people at the heart of the Ferrard programme are optimistic that a high quality statutory dementia service will continue, not withstanding the enormous expansion of private sector residential care homes and nursing homes which has taken place in Northern Ireland once Social Security funds became available to finance people entering private care. Although the expansion was slower to take off than in the rest of the United King-

dom, the growth has been extremely rapid as can be seen from the following table which refers to all client groups, not just people with dementia.

Number of Independent Sector Registered Homes

		Number of registered homes	Number of places
Residential Care Homes	1982	65	1416
	1987	131	2130
	1990	174	2904
Nursing Homes	1982	12	347
	1987	64	1564
	1990	164	5269
Total residential & nursing home beds			8173

Very few of these independent sector beds have been registered as beds for elderly mentally infirm people. It is however certain that some beds in both residential and nursing homes are occupied by people with varying degrees of cognitive impairment. It is not possible to say with any precision how many of the total 8,173 beds are actually occupied by people with moderate or severe dementia.

The Northern Board generally and the Bannside Unit of Management specifically are slowly reducing their direct provision of conventional residential beds for older people and are already contracting out services to the independent sector. In Bannside it is considered unlikely that the Board will withdraw from direct residential and community provision for mentally infirm people.

On the contrary, senior managers see the necessity for preserving and developing a strong active statutory dementia service. They see their skilled statutory staff continuing to be the leaders, teachers and demonstrators of good practice with this client group. They fervently believe that the skills and expertise needed to provide high quality service to people with dementia and their carers are acquired and upheld by continuing involvement in direct practice.

Having worked hard over many years to establish multi-disciplinary relationships and effective interweaving of formal and informal care, social services managers see

themselves as continuing to provide undisputed leadership in dementia services. As the statutory services assume responsibility for contracting and purchasing care, it is unlikely to be worth the independent sector's time in the immediate future to compete in the face of an openly declared determination to retain considerable statutory involvement in caring for vulnerable dementing people.

With the recent incorporation of the former Magherafelt/Cookstown region into the Bannside Unit of Management, demanding challenges lie ahead. Already the present pattern of service based on Ferrard is being replicated and refined in order to serve an area where virtually no service for people with dementia, other than home helps currently exists.

The coincidence of several organisational and structural changes have opened up new developmental opportunities. The realignment of new catchment areas for the psychiatric service through the implementation of the Donaldson Two plans, together with the change in social services boundaries and the release of funds linked to these changes, coupled with the retraction of psychiatric beds and a shrinking demand for conventional residential places have opened up new and exciting possibilities.

The future is certain to bring a much closer integration between social services and psychogeriatric services. The psychogeriatrician needs and wants to develop non-hospital alternatives for people in longstay psychogeriatric hospital beds. Social services wish to develop alternative residential type placements for the small number of people whose cognitive and behavioral deterioration makes them unsuitable for continued residence in Ferrard.

Both needs are likely to result in a plan which it is hoped will provide an improved quality of life for people who would otherwise have spent the rest of their lives in a continuing care ward of a psychiatric hospital. Plans are being actively pursued about developing an integrated statutory EMI residential-nursing home. It is likely that residential and nursing home services will be located in adjoining wings of a single building where domestic and day care services would be shared and each wing then managed as appropriate in order to meet the needs of its occupants. Joint assessment and respite care would

be facilitated and the unit would become the focus for community outreach.

It is envisaged that such a unit would be jointly funded with hospital retraction and social services funds and it would be jointly managed by nursing and social services staff. Residents could be easily transferred from one wing to another should their condition justify a transfer. If and when a transfer became necessary there would be the least possible disruption for the resident and their family.

Such a facility is unlikely to be a new build but more likely it will be an adaptation of an existing conventional residential home. The best aspects of the Ferrard approach to care will be maintained and nursing elements will be grafted on.

If such plans come to fruition there should be no need for anyone with dementia, even in the most advanced stage of the disease to be admitted to a psychiatric hospital. Such visionary plans mean that a continuing major responsibility for this client group is likely to be retained by the statutory health and social services. Much professional effort and considerable financial resources will continue to be expended on sustaining people in the community for as long as their social functioning, health and the wellbeing of their carers permits. Then there will be a range of residential and nursing home provision situated near to their home communities committed to meeting dependency needs in a stimulating high quality caring environment in so far as human expertise and financial resources permit.

Knowledge of the incidence, etiology and treatment of dementing illnesses will not stand still. Neither will the creative imaginative response of the Health and Social Services staff of the Bannside Unit of Management of the Northern Health and Social Services Board.

REFERENCES

Allen, I. in Judge, K. and Sinclair, I. (eds.) (1986) *Residential Care For Elderly People.*

Burnside, I. (1984) *Working With the Elderly Group Process and Techniques,* California, Wadsworth.

CPA. (1990) *Community Life: a Code of Practice for Community Care,* London, CPA.

Department of Health. (1989) *Working For Patients,* London, HMSO.

Department of Health. (1989) *Caring for People,* London: HMSO.

Department of Health Social Services Inspectorate. (1989) *Homes Are For Living In,* London, HMSO.

DHSS (NI). (1986) *A Regional Strategy for Northern Ireland Health and Personal Social Services,* Belfast, HMSO.

DHSS (NI). (1990) *People First: Community Care in Northern Ireland,* Belfast, HMSO.

Godlove, C. Richard, L. & Rodwell, G. (1982) *Time For Action,* Sheffield, Joint Unit for Social Services Research University of Sheffield.

Department of Health. (1989) *Caring for Patients,* London, HMSO.

Maslow, A. (1954) *Motivation and Personality,* New York, Harper and Row.

Miller, E. & Gwynne, G. (1974) *A Life Apart,* London, Tavistock.

Miller, J. (1991) 'Thanks for the memory,' *Social Work Today,* 25 April. 14–15.

Norman, A. (1987) *Severe Dementia: the Provision of Longstay Care,* London: CPA.

Seligman, M. (1974) Depression and learned helplessness in Friedman, R. & Katz, M. (eds.) *Psychology of Depression: Contemporary Theory and Research,* New York, Halstead.

Wagner, G. (1988) *A Positive Choice Report of the Independent Review of Residential Care,* London, NISW.

Wright, F. (1991) 'A Home From Home', *Social Work Today,* 25 April. 34–35.

'FERRARD' ASSESSMENT SCHEDULE	
RESIDENT'S NAME .... DATE OF BIRTH .... DATE OF ADMISSION	
MOBILITY	*BATHING*
DRESSING	*USE OF TOILET*
FEEDING	*CONTINENCE*

APPENDIX 1

'FERRARD' ASSESSMENT SCHEDULE

RESIDENT'S NAME .... DATE OF BIRTH .... DATE OF ADMISSION ....

ORIENTATION	*SLEEPING*
COMMUNICATION	*SOCIAL RELATIONS*
CONCENTRATION	*MEMORY*

| NAME .... DATE OF ADMISSION .... |
| DATE OF BIRTH .... |

PROBLEMS OF ACTIVITIES OF DAILY LIVING	OBJECTIVES OF CARE	PLAN OF CARE
PHYSICAL		
SOCIAL		
BEHAVIOURAL		
SLEEP PATTERN		

69

DAILY LIVING FACT SHEET

Name of Resident : _____   Unit : _____

ROUTINE ON WAKING

Requires to be taken to the toilet ☐

Prefers to use commode ☐

Requires help with washing ☐

Can wash self ☐

Requires help with dressing ☐

Can dress self ☐

Likes to remain in own room ☐

Prefers to go to sitting room ☐

BEDTIME ROUTINE

Enjoys bath in the evening ☐

Number of pillows ☐

Likes dentures removed ☐

Sleeps well ☐

Needs sedation ☐

Sleeps with night light ☐

Requires bedroom door open ☐

BREAKFAST/LUNCH/DINNER

Small appetite ☐

Good appetite ☐

No known dislikes ☐

Requires assistance ☐

Requires special diet ☐

Specify – liquidised ☐

    – diabetic ☐

    – gastric ☐

    – low fat ☐

DAILY ACTIVITIES

Shopping ☐

Visits to friends ☐

Rests ☐

TV ☐

Radio ☐

Music ☐

Painting ☐

Knitting ☐

Crafts ☐

Gardens ☐

Reading ☐

LIKES/DISLIKES & ANY KNOWN ALLERGIES

SPECIFY :	LIKES	DIS-LIKES
Fruit		
Vegetables		
Meat		
Poultry		
Fish		
Beverages		
Condiments		
Cigarettes		
Alcohol		
Reading material		

KNOWN ALLERGIES: _____

RELIGIOUS OBSERVANCE FORBIDS: _____

GENERAL HEALTH

State of Health – Good ☐
         – Frail

Eyesight – Good ☐
    – Poor

Wear Glasses [YES] [NO]

Hearing – Good ☐
    – Poor

PREFERRED BEDTIME DRINKS

Horlicks ☐   Ovaltine ☐
Chocolate ☐   Cocoa ☐
Tea ☐   Coffee ☐

PHYSICAL HEALTH

Special Drugs, e.g.

Iron   Insulin   Others
☐   ☐   ☐

DETAILS _____

_____

_____

Takes liquid medicine in tea ☐
Tablets crushed in food ☐

SENSITIVITY TO DRUGS – OTHERS

_____

REQUIRES AID FOR WALKING (Specify)

_____

_____

PERSONAL HYGIENE

Interested & cares about appearance ☐
Bathes AM   PM ☐
Wears dentures ☐
Pedicure – Regular care given ☐
Hairdresser – Regular ☐
Shampoo and set ☐
Perms ☐
Hair not cut – Religious beliefs ☐
Special Help needed with –
Requires assistance with
general toilette ☐

GENERAL HEALTH (Contd)

DISABILITY

INCONTINENCE

Urine ☐   Faeces ☐

*ACTIVITIES, OCCUPATIONS, LINKS
WITH THE COMMUNITY*

Member of Society, Group Organisation

_____

Active Church Goer _____

Others _____

Favourite regular outdoor activity

_____

Favourite TV Programmes

_____

Favourite Radio Programmes _____

_____

Type of Music liked _____

Day Trips ☐
Concerts ☐
Walks ☐
Bingo ☐

SOCIAL NEEDS & RELATIONSHIPS

Enjoys meeting others ☐
Opportunity to discover their
interests and skills ☐
Discuss pattern of their lives ☐
Expects basic right for privacy
as an emotional need ☐
Expects not to need to conceal
emotions ☐
Expects to be denied emotional
or sexual needs ☐
Expects not to be discouraged
from forming close personal
relationships ☐

71

TERMINAL CARE

Last Rites and Counselling _____
_____

Minister/Priest/Counsellor

Name _____

Telephone Number _____

Personal Wishes, e.g. Family, Friends in
Attendance etc

_____
_____
_____

FUNERAL ARRANGEMENTS

Person Responsible

Name _____

Telephone Number _____

REQUESTS

Private _____

Wreaths, Flowers etc _____

Cremation _____

Burial _____

Expand _____

_____
_____

SOCIAL NEEDS & RELATIONSHIPS
(Contd)

Enjoys talking about early family life	
Can relate family history	
Can keep up to date with family relationships, Births, Deaths etc	
Keeps contact with long standing friends	
Feels it is important to discuss bereavement of family, friends	

Mr. and Mrs. Brown live in a three bedroom Housing Executive house on the outskirts of Antrim town. Mr. Brown originally came from Belfast and Mrs. Brown from Larne. She is the youngest of a family of six, four brothers and one sister are now deceased. Mrs. Brown attended primary school in Antrim and on leaving school at 14 years of age her family moved to Belfast for work. She worked as a spinner in the York Street Spinning Company which manufactured linen from raw flax. At the outbreak of the Second World War her family returned to Antrim. She had already met her future husband while living in Belfast and they married when she was 24 years of age.

Mrs. Brown gave up work when she married and had only one daughter who emigrated to Australia some time ago. The couple have had a close relationship over the years and until recently were able to go everywhere together. They celebrated their golden wedding recently and have never been separated.

Mrs. Brown is a well built 74 year old lady. She has thinning grey hair, wears glasses and is usually tidy in appearance. According to Mr. Brown his wife in the past would have been a pleasant, outgoing lady whose interests were sewing, knitting, walking, crocheting, baking and she was also solo singer in their local church choir. Since 1988 he has found his wife's personality greatly changed. From this date she would sit by the fire looking very dour and solemn or wander about the kitchen attempting to place dishes or pots inappropriately on the cooker. Mr. Brown has stated that his wife would constantly have given him menacing looks and also looked in this manner to any visitors to their home. Mrs. Brown continued to be uncooperative with her husband and became disorientated in time and place. By 1989 Mrs. Brown frequently had disturbed nights and she would wander downstairs and it was at this time she became incontinent of urine by day and night.

Mr. Brown became very concerned about his wife's deteriorating condition and Mrs. Brown was assessed in February 1989 by Dr. Compton, Psychogeriatrican and was diagnosed as suffering from Alzheimers's Disease. Dr. Compton provided advice and guidance at this stage.

There was a noticeable deterioration in Mrs. Brown's condition since then. Her dependence on her husband increased and she required full assistance with daily living skills i.e. dressing/undressing, feeding, toileting. There were times when she became unsteady on her feet and required supervision when walking, particularly when transferring on and off a chair, bed or toilet. She had great difficulty at meal times and was unaware of how to use her cutlery.

Mr. Brown is a slightly built man who is experiencing great difficulty with his wife's lack of mobility. In March 1989 he accepted support provided by the Domiciliary worker from Ferrard House EMI Unit who commenced a planned programme of care. Through multi-disciplinary assessment the Occupational Therapist was contacted re requirements for the Browns such as aids and adaptations. Social Services fitted a stairway hand rail and rails on either side of the toilet to assist Mrs. Brown's mobility. Negotiations are still ongoing from this date with the Housing Executive re-structuring the bathroom by removing the bath and fitting a walk-in shower stall. Because of Mrs. Brown's wandering during the night a sensory door pad was provided for the entrance to their bedroom. Mr. Brown's deafness prevented him always hearing when his wife got up and wandered at night and the security he received from knowing the buzzer by his bed would waken him, enabled him to get some sleep at night.

Mr. Brown had been informed by the Domiciliary worker of Outreach Services available at Ferrard House, but it wasn't until he realised he could no longer cope with his wife's incontinence that his reluctance to use them ceased. In June 1990 he accepted a service provided by the Geriatric Service and received a supply of incontinent pads every fortnight. He also availed of the Home Help Service and received meals on wheels every Tuesday and Thursday. During the last six months of 1990, Mrs. Brown continued to deteriorate. She had become quite aggressive in manner and when Mr. Brown attempted to assist her with daily living skills she became hostile and resisted his help. On occasions she would strike out attempting to hit her husband.

At this time Mr. Brown agreed to use Ferrard Day Care facilities and initially brought his wife on Mondays and Fridays to the unit. He quite often used the luncheon club in Ferrard while he visited friends or shopped. On several occasions he used the 'Sitting Service' the unit provides when he went to Dublin to collect visitors from America during the month of September. The change in Mrs. Brown's personality saddens Mr. Brown as he maintained it was so uncharacteristic of how she was in past days.

Initially Mr. Brown was opposed to accepting Respite Care in Ferrard House as his aim had been to maintain his wife's care in their home. However, since accepting Day Care in Ferrard he had become familiar with unit staff and the confidence he achieved enabled him to accept respite care for one week in October 1990. This may have lessened his initial reservation regarding respite care but it was an extremely difficult decision to make and Mr. Brown continued to be very emotional at the thought of his wife being separated from him.

During this week in Ferrard when he visited his wife every day, with staff encouragement he decided to attend the Family Support Group's monthly meeting and was agreeably surprised to find it very supportive. He has said that he found it a relief to know that other carers had experienced similar feelings and pressures as himself. Mr. Brown acknowledged that his exhaustion, weight loss and pale complexion were probably due to the stress he experienced in trying to care for his wife at home. On return to her home Mrs. Brown's behavioural problems increased and Mr. Brown found it increasingly more difficult to care for his wife. He again requested Respite Care in December 1990 and Mrs. Brown was admitted to Ferrard on 15th December.

From that date Mrs. Brown has occupied a respite bed, has settled well in the unit and is managed by the use of a daily, varied, activity group therapy programme of care. She is now continent of urine which was established by maintaining a 2 hourly, toileting programme. Her sleep pattern has been re-established and Mrs. Brown presents no management problems. She frequently plays the piano during musical entertainment and therapy sessions for other residents and also at the Wednesday evening friendship club.

This continuum of care experience has made approaching the subject of permanent care a little less difficult for Mr. Brown.

Prior to the present period of respite care he had always refused to consider permanent care and although he still remains very emotional at this prospect, seeing this as a final parting from his wife, he now states that perhaps this may be the best course of action for both of them.

He has been assured that he may continue in his role as 'caring husband' and is welcome in the unit at anytime. He is now involved in discussion with his wife's primary worker and team leader.

Mr. Brown applied for permanent admission to care for his wife on 16th January 1991 and this process will be completed and a permanent bed offered to Mrs. Brown at the multi-disciplinary admission panel meeting later this month. Meantime Mr. Brown's health improves and he is presently preparing a scrapbook of his wife's life history using anecdotes and photographs to assist Ferrard staff during Reality Orientation and Reminiscence work to maintain Mrs. Brown's present level of functioning.

APPENDIX 4

Session	Monday	Tuesday	Wednesday	Thursday	Friday	Saturday	Sunday	Groups
10.30 AM	**Group B** Daily News and Current Affairs	**Group C** Daily News with Current Affairs	**Group B** Poetry for Reminiscence	**Group C** Art Therapy and Crafts1	Hair Dressing with on-going individual therapy i.e. walks shopping outings visiting — Seasonal Activities — Personal Preference Activities	**Group B** Sing-a-long and Dancing	Morning Worship	A Day Care
To 11.30 AM	**Group C** Story-telling with Reminiscence	**Group B** RO with Reminiscence	**Group C** Music and Movement for Stimulation	**Group B** Daily News with Story-telling		**Group C** Happy Hour	One to One Visitors	B
2.30 PM	**Group D** RO and Reminiscence	**Group D** Music and Movement for Stimulation	**Group D** Story-telling for Reminiscence	**Group D** Sing-a-long Session		**Group D** Poetry and RO	Music for Relaxation	C
To 3.30 PM	**Group B** Art Therapy	Or Join All Groups Interdenom-inational Church Service	**Group B** Music for Relaxation	**Group C** Story-telling with Reminiscence		**Group B** Happy Hour	Video and Film Choices	D
EVENINGS	THE FRIENDSHIP CLUB EACH WEDNESDAY EVENING AT ALL TIMES FACILITATE COMMUNICATION AND DEVELOP HOME ORIENTATION WITH 24 HOUR REALITY ORIENTATION FERRARD — DAILY GROUP THERAPY ACTIVITY IDENTIFICATION							

CLIENTS PERSONAL FILE

NAME: _____

ADDRESS: _____

_____

DATE OF BIRTH: _____

RELIGION: _____

FAMILY DOCTOR: _____

ADDRESS: _____

_____

TELEPHONE NO: _____

NEXT OF KIN: _____

RELATIONSHIP: _____

ADDRESS: _____

_____

TELEPHONE NO: _____

SOCIAL WORKER: _____

FIELDWORK OFFICE: _____

_____

ANY OTHER INFORMATION: _____

_____

_____

_____

_____

_____

APPENDIX 6

SESSIONS	MONDAY	TUESDAY	WEDNESDAY	THURSDAY	FRIDAY	DAY CARE
9.30 AM	Daily News Current Affairs RO	Daily News Current Affairs RO	Daily News Current Affairs RO	Daily News Current Affairs RO	Hairdressing	
10.30 AM	Morning Tea and Self Help Skills Tidy Up Kitchen	Morning Tea and Self Help Skills Tidy Up Kitchen	Morning Tea and Self Help Skills Tidy Up Kitchen	Morning Tea and Self Help Skills Tidy Up Kitchen		
11.15 AM	Craft	Art	Reminiscence	Cookery		
12.00 Noon	Personal Hygiene	Personal Hygiene	Personal Hygiene	Personal Hygiene	Personal Hygiene	
12.30 PM	LUNCH	LUNCH	LUNCH	LUNCH	LUNCH	
1.30 PM to 2.30 PM	Reminiscence with Poetry	Interdenomin-ational Church Service in the Unit	Musical Movement To Tapes	Games	On-going Individual Therapy i.e. Walks Shopping	
	Afternoon Tea Self Help Skills	Afternoon Tea Self Help Skills	Afternoon Tea Self Help Skills	Afternoon Tea Self Help Skills		
3.00 PM to 3.45 PM	General Conversation	Return to Day Care Sing-a-long	Bathing of Day Care members	Reminiscence with music or slides	Seasonal Activities	
	Preparation for Tea served in unit i.e. personal hygiene	Preparation for Tea served in unit i.e. personal hygiene	Preparation for Tea served in unit i.e. personal hygiene	Preparation for Tea served in unit i.e. personal hygiene	Preparation for Tea i.e. personal hygiene	
	FERRARD DAY CARE CENTRE GROUP THERAPY ACTIVITY IDENTIFICATION					

Activities   50
Admission, criteria   23
Admission, process   24, 59
Allen, I.   59, 66
Antrim/Ballymena   7, 9, 20, 54
Art   50
Assessment   14, 32, 34
Assessment instruments   23
Assessment Schedule,
   Ferrard   24, 67, 68, 69
Bathing   29, 30, 31
Birthdays and celebrations   38
Burnside, I.   33, 66
Cape   10, 24
Care plan   69
Care staff, duties   18
Carers support group   54, 55, 60
Caring For People   8
Case study   73
Centre for Policy on Ageing   66
Chiropody   59
Choice   34, 35, 36, 37, 60
Clothing   36
Club   45, 47, 51, 58, 75
Community psychiatric nurse   57
Confidentiality   18, 27, 28
Continence management   5, 24, 30
Continuum of care   75
DHSS   4, 9
Daily living fact sheet   24, 70, 71, 72
Day care   34, 48, 52
Day care application form   77
Day care programme   48, 50
Day Centre   12
Death   19, 34
Department of Health   4, 66
Design   11
Dignity   28
Domestic activities   48, 50
Domestic staff   13
Domiciliary care   53

Domiciliary worker   14, 48, 49,
   53, 54, 57, 60, 73, 74
Drugs   39
Financial arrangements   41
Food   37, 38
Free Funds   34, 60
Friendship club   45, 47, 58, 75
Fulfilment   43
Furnishings   11
Garden   39
Godlove, C.   33, 66
Group work   45, 50
Gwynne, G.   43, 66
Hairdressing   29
Homes Are for Living In   9
Independence   32, 33, 34, 35
Induction, staff   15, 18
In-house group work programme   45
In-service training   15, 18, 19
Inter-disciplinary work   57
Judge, K.   66
Key worker   39, 44
Laundry service   34, 36, 55, 57
Lunch club   55, 58, 74
Magherafelt/Cookstown   7, 9, 14, 63
Management staff   15, 18
Maslow, A.   43, 66
Medical care   39
Meals   37, 38
Miller, E.   21, 43, 66
Miller, J.   66
Mobility   23
Multi-disciplinary team   20, 24, 57, 63
Music   46, 50
Norman, A.   7, 8, 16, 66
Nursing homes, private   40, 62
Objectives, Ferrard   10, 49
Outings   39
People First   8, 40, 62, 66
Personal appearance   29
Primary worker   17, 29, 35

Privacy   26, 28, 34, 36, 41
Private sector   40, 62
Psychogeriatrician   5, 20, 21,
   24, 25, 30, 31, 39, 53, 64, 73
Records   15, 27
Regional strategy   8
Rehabilitation   7, 52
Relatives, support   34, 51
Religion   42
Reminiscence   46, 48, 50, 75
Residential care   9, 34, 35, 52
Residents, characteristics   32,
   33, 35, 36, 38
Respite care   34, 48, 57, 58, 64, 74, 75
Review process   27
Richard, L.   33, 66
Rights   27, 40, 41, 42, 43
Rodwell, G.   33, 66
Security   26, 27, 32
Seligman, M.   32, 66
Senior care staff, duties   16, 17, 18, 20
Shared care, see respite
   care   34, 48, 57, 58, 64, 74, 75
Sinclair, I.   66
Social Services Inspectorate   4, 9, 66
Social workers   27, 53
Staffing establishment   13
Staff training, see in-service
   training   7
Supervision, staff   20, 32
Support group   5, 33, 55
Training, see in-service training   18
Twenty four hour help line   56
Unit of Management   7, 9, 14,
   18, 34, 63, 65
Voluntary organisation   47
Volunteers   47
Wagner, G.   9, 32, 66
Wandering   32
Working for Patients   8
Wright, F.   66

Printed in the United Kingdom for HMSO
Dd 302996   C30   11/91   55-8976   29254